Food Poisoning

By G. M. DACK, M.D.

Revised and Enlarged

THE UNIVERSITY OF CHICAGO PRESS

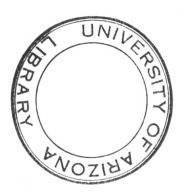

Library of Congress Catalog Number: 55-12510

THE UNIVERSITY OF CHICAGO PRESS, CHICAGO 37
Cambridge University Press, London, N.W. 1, England
The University of Toronto Press, Toronto 5, Canada

© *1943, 1949, and 1956 by The University of Chicago.*
Published 1956. Composed and printed by THE UNIVER-
SITY OF CHICAGO PRESS, *Chicago, Illinois, U.S.A.*

Food Poisoning

This book is dedicated to the memory
of my colleague and friend William E. Cary

Preface to the Third Edition

Since the publication of the last edition of *Food Poisoning*, progress involving all classes of causative agents has been made in the entire field of food poisoning. The problem of chemical additives to foods has received increased emphasis in our law-enforcement agencies. New material has been added in this book on plant and animal poisons in foods. The portion dealing with bacterial food poisoning has been increased and extensively revised.

The author is particularly indebted to his colleagues, who, through their research, have contributed knowledge to the field of food poisoning. An effort has been made to bring the book up to date by the revision of all chapters.

The author is indebted to Dr. Bruce W. Halstead for his assistance concerning fish poisoning. For the aid from his colleagues, Dr. Michael J. Surgalla, Dr. Merlin S. Bergdoll, Dr. Hiroshi Sugiyama, and Dr. Raphael O. Wagenaar, he is especially indebted. To Dr. Charles F. Niven, Jr., who has helped with the chapters on *Staphylococcus* and *Streptococcus faecalis*, the author is appreciative. The author is especially obligated to Dr. Lloyd B. Jensen, who has read and made suggestions on all chapters. This revision would not have been possible without the kind assistance in editing and preparation of the manuscript by Miss Ruth Laser and Mrs. Patricia Christiansen.

G. M. DACK

Preface to the Second Edition

The useful purpose which this little book has served during and after World War II has been gratifying beyond expectation to its author. The problems of processing and distributing food during the war added to our knowledge of food poisoning; hence an attempt has been made to bring the subject matter up to date, and, in so doing, the author has indebted himself to many friends and colleagues. Among those to whom reference is not made in the text are Mr. Hiroshi Sugiyama for his help in revising the chapter on botulism, Dr. Michael Surgalla for assistance with the chapter on staphylococcus food poisoning, Dr. Elizabeth Verder and Dr. Morris D. Schneider for their help in revising the chapter on *Salmonella*, and Dr. Charles Niven, Jr., for his assistance in revising the chapter on α-type streptococci in relation to food poisoning. Dr. K. Eileen Hite has read many portions of the revision and offered helpful criticism. Miss Joan Kadavy has been especially helpful in checking the Bibliography. The author is particularly indebted to his secretary, Miss Shirley Ann Kenney, whose tireless efforts have made this revision possible.

G. M. DACK

Preface to the First Edition

The term "food poisoning" is, of necessity, vague. Properly included in this category are illnesses resulting from ingestion of food containing certain inorganic chemicals, poisons derived from animals and plants, and toxic products or infections caused by several species of bacteria. Exact characterization of these disorders, produced by such a diverse group of inciting agents, is impossible because they do not present a uniform syndrome and are therefore variously classified by different authors.

Perhaps the most characteristic feature of an outbreak of food poisoning is the explosive nature of the illness, which is generally characterized by gastrointestinal upsets. There are, however, important exceptions, such as, for example, botulism, in which the gastrointestinal symptoms are generally a minor feature of the disease.

In the present book I have included the following causative agents: chemicals, poisonous plants and animals, bacteria and their products, viruses, protozoans, helminths, and a miscellaneous group of illnesses, the causes of which are unknown. Of this list, the bacteria which form toxins in food before ingestion are discussed at greatest length. Botulism and staphylococcus food poisoning, which are induced by toxins preformed in the food, represent the more typical diseases in this classification. The gastrointestinal upsets associated with the *Salmonella* infections should be considered more strictly as food-borne infections, although they are universally classified as food poisoning.

It is a pleasure to acknowledge my indebtedness to many friends and associates for invaluable aid in my work in this field during the last twenty years. I am indebted to Professor F. W. Tanner, under whose direction my interest in food poisoning was aroused; to the late Professor E. O. Jordan, with whom I was associated as student and colleague; and to other associates with whom I worked at various times, in particular to Professor W. A. Starin, Drs. W. E. Cary,

Willard Wood, James Gibbard, Oram C. Woolpert, Ellen Davison, and Milton Segalove.

I am indebted to Professors W. H. Taliaferro and R. W. Harrison and to Dr. Ellen Davison for help in preparing this book, and I am especially indebted to Mrs. W. H. Taliaferro for revising the manuscript.

G. M. Dack

Table of Contents

I Introduction

During the last century, changes have taken place in man's mode of living that have brought about new methods of processing and preparing foods. The modern age of invention has created specialization in industry, so that the individual is no longer called upon to produce his own food. With modern transportation and refrigeration, fresh fruits and vegetables are grown in favorable areas and shipped, either canned or fresh, to distant markets. This applies to the canning or handling of fresh meats. Experience has shown that food-poisoning problems may arise when new procedures are instituted in preparing and storing foods.

Although food poisoning may result from a diverse group of inciting agents, there is still a tendency to disguise the causative agent under the blanket term "ptomaine" poisoning. This term has been used popularly since its introduction in 1870 by Selmi, the Italian toxicologist. "Ptomaine" was taken from the word *ptoma,* meaning "corpse." There is neither a specific entity nor a group of substances which can be properly called "ptomaine"; therefore, the term is unscientific and meaningless.

There is a popular tendency to associate food poisoning with putrefaction. It is now known that putrefaction in a food does not necessarily give rise to the toxic substances involved in food poisoning. An example of a wholesome food containing putrefactive bacteria and their products is Limburger cheese. Other examples are rotten seal meat and fish eaten by the Eskimos in Greenland, rotten fish used by the Samoyedes, and rotten eggs served by the Chinese (1).[1] Many peoples of the world consider rotten meat a delicacy. Another case in point is food contaminated with *Clostridium sporogenes,* one of the most putrefactive of bacteria. Cultures of this bacterium have been repeatedly fed to experimental animals without producing any evidence of illness. Furthermore, these cultures have been injected intraperitoneally and intravenously without causing ill

1. All references will be found at the end of each chapter.

1

effects. As a matter of fact, cultures of *Cl. sporogenes* were used in World War I to treat suppurative war wounds, with reported beneficial effects (2).

INVESTIGATION OF FOOD-POISONING OUTBREAKS

Small outbreaks of gastrointestinal upsets occurring in the family are usually not reported. In general, no recognition is given the event, and the family physician is seldom summoned. When several people are affected who may have attended the same banquet or eaten at the same public eating establishment, considerable attention is given the episode by health authorities and the press. Illnesses in small family groups due to the fatal type of food poisoning known as "botulism" are usually reported, but this type of food poisoning is uncommon.

Small family outbreaks which do become known are generally brought to light through complaints made by a member of the family to the grocer or butcher in connection with a suspected item of food. In the majority of cases the complaint is not carried further, although reports are sometimes made by the retailer to the manufacturer or producer, and these, in most instances, are investigated. Much time often elapses between the illness and the investigation, thus making it difficult or impossible to determine the causative agent. Frequently, meat is suspected by the family as the cause, since it agrees with the false "ptomaine" notion of food poisoning. In many cases, upon investigation, the food item alleged to be responsible for an outbreak is exonerated, and another item of food or some other cause is found.

One of the distinctive characteristics of an outbreak of food poisoning is the sudden illness of several individuals following a specific meal at which a definite item of food is implicated. Often only one person in such a group develops gastrointestinal symptoms. Some of these cases of one illness are actually brought to court for trial. The alleged symptoms are one or more of the following: nausea, vomiting, diarrhea, and abdominal cramping. Careful study of the individuals often reveals one of a large variety of other illnesses; coronary heart or gall-bladder disease, passage of renal calculi, appendicitis, brain tumors, certain forms of intestinal allergy, cerebral hemorrhage, onset of infectious diseases, and functional bowel distress associated with emotional upsets may be causing the symptoms. Local chilling of the abdomen (caused by sleeping uncovered) has been reported to give rise to many cases of acute nonspecific diarrhea (3). This phenomenon was observed in World War II among military personnel stationed in hot climates.

It is important after an outbreak of food poisoning that it be immediately investigated if the true cause is to be established. A delay of hours after vomiting and diarrhea may mean that chemical poisons have been discarded in the vomitus and excreta. If none of the original food remains, it may be difficult to identify the specific agent. In food poisoning of bacterial origin, a delay of hours may often bring about marked bacterial changes in a perishable product which were not present at the time of consumption. From a legal standpoint, a prompt and intelligent investigation may prevent unnecessary litigation and provide the basis for a fair settlement if settlement appears warranted. It is generally important to ascertain what items of food were eaten at previous meals for a period of 48 hours. When a large number of cases occur within as short a period as 2–3 hours after eating, attention should be centered on the last meal and on any food eaten by a majority of the persons afflicted. When the onset of symptoms in various individuals appears over a period of many hours, it is important to know the items of food in the diet for several previous meals. If the outbreak involves persons who have shared a particular meal or eaten at one place, it is a good plan to prepare a list of the various items of food served and check these items with persons who ate the meal or who ate at the place in question. Frequently, a single item may be found to be the common denominator for those who are made ill. If this fact is observed, time may be saved by having a laboratory examination made directly on the incriminated food item. Usually, not every individual will be made ill when a specific item is involved. Such variables as the amount eaten (dosage) and individual resistance play an important part. Generally, however, the majority of people partaking of the involved food will be affected when such an outbreak occurs. Sometimes psychic disturbances account for symptoms in some individuals who are present during the illness of others but who may not have eaten the incriminated food. If too long a time elapses before the investigation is started, the data obtainable are less reliable, for many people find it difficult to remember what they have eaten or whether they experienced any symptoms at the time in question. An excellent questionnaire has been prepared by individuals concerned with the investigation of food-poisoning outbreaks. These forms are reproduced here.

[FORM 1]

QUESTIONS FOR PERSONS ALLEGING ILLNESS FROM FOOD

1. What is the name?_____Age?_____
2. Address?_____
3. Are you employed in any business and, if so, by whom?_____
_____
4. Married or single?_____
5. How long after eating were you made ill?_____
6. Were others made ill?_____If so, who? (Age of each?)_____
_____
7. Did any person eat the same foods without becoming ill?_____
8. If so, who? (Names and addresses?)_____
_____
9. What were the first symptoms of your illness and when did they occur?_____
_____
10. Was there pain in the stomach or abdomen?_____
_____
11. Was there vomiting?_____For how long?_____
12. Was there diarrhea or constipation?_____
13. Please tell anything else you remember about your illness and the events leading up to it:_____
_____
_____
_____
_____
_____
14. How long did the acute illness last?_____
15. Please itemize expenses, if any, resulting from your illness:_____
_____
16. What is the name and address of the doctor who attended you during your illness?_____
_____
17. Is he your regular doctor?_____If not, who is?_____
_____
18. When were you last attended by a doctor before this illness and for what cause?_____

19. Have you ever undergone an operation and, if so, for what?_____

20. Have you had stomach or digestive trouble in the past?_____
21. If so, of what nature?_____

22. To what did the doctor attribute the illness?_____

23. Do you attribute the illness to the eating of any particular food?_____

24. If so, what food?_____

25. Why?_____
26. What foods did you eat at the suspected meal?_____

27. What was eaten at the four meals preceding the suspected meal? (All foods eaten at each meal, if possible, and also between meals.)

_____

_____

_____

28. What foods, if any, did you eat between the suspected meal and the onset of your illness?_____

29. Did the doctor take the container or any of the suspected food left after the meal?_____
30. Did you feed any of the suspected food to dogs, chickens, or other animals?_____

    If so, were they made sick?_____
31. Have you the container or any portion of the foods which you believe caused the illness?_____
32. If not, what was done with them?_____

33. From whom was food purchased and by whom?_____

_____

34. Date of purchase:_____
35. Give name of brand and or manufacturer or distributor on label:_____

36. Did you ask for that particular brand?_____
37. Are you accustomed to buying that particular brand?_____
38. Where was the food left before using?_____
39. Where was the food kept after unwrapping or opening?_____

40. State as exactly as possible how the food was prepared and served:

_____

_____

41. Did the appearance or odor indicate anything unusual in the food on unwrapping or opening? _____
If so, please give particulars: _____
_____

42. On what date and at what meal was the food eaten? _____

43. At the time of eating the food, did you notice any peculiarity in the appearance, taste, or odor of it? _____ If so, please describe:
_____
_____

Witness: _____   _____
Date: _____ 195 _____   [*Signature*]

[FORM 2]

QUESTIONS FOR THE ATTENDING PHYSICIAN
IN CASE OF ALLEGED ILLNESS

1. Name and address of physician: _____
_____
2. Name of patient: _____
3. On what date or dates did you treat this patient? _____
_____
4. How long had the patient been ill when you arrived? _____
_____
5. Was the onset of the disease sudden, or had there been previous illness? _____
6. How many persons were ill of the same type of disease and under your observation? _____
7. What were the general symptoms (appearance of patient, continuous or spasmodic pains, nervous, excited, or in coma, vomiting, or diarrhea)? _____
_____
8. What was the pulse rate? _____
9. Regular or intermittent? _____
10. Pulse tension? _____
11. Was the temperature persistently above or below normal? _____
12. What were the highest and lowest points reached? _____
13. Was a temperature and pulse record kept? _____
14. What was the number of respirations per minute and character?
_____
15. Was there any disturbance of vision? _____
16. What disturbance of the reflexes, if any, was noted? _____
_____
_____
17. How long did the attack continue? _____
18. General remarks: _____
_____
_____

19. Was any bacteriological or chemical examination made of the blood, vomitus, or excreta?_____

20. What was your diagnosis?_____

21. If food poisoning, what food do you believe caused the illness?

_____

22. Was a laboratory examination made of any suspected food?_____

23. If so, what was found?_____

24. What treatment was followed or prescribed?_____

_____

25. Was any morphine or opiate used to alleviate pain?_____

26. Was any strychnine or other stimulant used?_____

27. Do you consider recovery complete?_____

_____

28. Have you a detailed record of the case?_____

29. Have you attended this patient before?_____If so, for what ailment?_____

In case of death:

30. Was an autopsy performed or any post mortem specimens examined?

_____

31. If so, by whom was such autopsy or examination made?_____

_____

*Witness:*_____   _____

*Date:*_____*195*_____   [*Signature*]

When the investigator has obtained the necessary information, it is generally possible to get a clue to the agent involved, so that treatment of the patient may be begun immediately. Furthermore, if a specific agent is suspected, time is saved in the laboratory tests. The problem of determining whether the agent is chemical, plant, or animal poison, bacterial toxins, or a food-borne infection is often difficult. The solution is simplified by a careful field investigation. Reference to Tables 1, 2, and 13 and to the following résumé of some of the general points for differentiating the causative agents will prove helpful in this regard. A more complete account of the specific agents is detailed in subsequent chapters. The final diagnosis in all instances is made in the laboratory.

Chemical poisoning.—In general, chemical poisoning is characterized by a short interval of time elapsing between the swallowing of a poisonous food and the onset of the symptoms. This lapse may vary from 10 minutes to 2 hours. An exception to the short incubation period is methyl alcohol poisoning, where symptoms usually develop 18–48 hours after ingestion, although occasional transitory symptoms may occur within 1 hour. The history of the outbreak may suggest the specific chemical. For example, antimony poisoning has occurred from eating foods cooked in cheap, gray-enameled cooking utensils. Cadmium poisoning is usually associated with acid liquids in cadmium-plated metal utensils. These two chemical poisons give rise to vomiting, cramps, and diarrhea about $\frac{1}{2}$ hour after eating. Sodium fluoride poisoning should be considered if this insecticide is used in the kitchen, because it is often mistaken for baking powder, soda, or flour. In addition to vomiting, cramps, and diarrhea occurring within a few minutes to 2 hours after eating, paresis of certain groups of muscles may occur and suggest sodium fluoride. Acute poisoning due to arsenic, lead, or mercury is not usually associated with foods except where these chemicals have been added maliciously. However, lead and arsenic used in sprays and alkaloids should be taken into account.

Poisonous plants or animals.—The nature of poisoning from plants and animals is varied. Mussel poisoning is suggested if mussels from the Pacific Coast are eaten at particular seasons of the year. Symptoms of respiratory paralysis with the loss of power in the muscles of the extremities and neck would also suggest mussel poisoning. Favism is associated with eating or being in the vicinity of the fava bean when it is in blossom. (This plant is widely cultivated in this country by people of Italian extraction.) The symptoms are acute febrile anemia, with jaundice, hematuria, and hemoglobinuria. Snakeroot poisoning is characterized by a slower onset of symptoms and a history of drinking milk from cows pastured in wooded areas where snakeroot is abundant. The symptoms are weakness, prostration, pernicious vomiting, and severe constipation. Mushroom poisoning is apparent 6–15 hours after eating poisonous varieties of mushrooms. It is characterized by hypoglycemia and convulsions, severe abdominal pain, intense thirst, nausea, retching, and vomiting, with profuse watery evacuations. Ergotism is rare in this country and is associated with eating meal or bread made from rye contaminated with the fungus *Claviceps purpurea*. Water-hemlock poisoning is uncommon and usually occurs when the leaves or roots of this plant are eaten by mistake. In some parts of the world honey has been implicated in food poisoning and has been associated with specific flowers from which the bees gather nectar. During World War I rhubarb leaves were recommended as a substitute for greens, and many cases of oxalate poisoning resulted. It is obvious that the symptoms derived from eating poisonous plants or animals may vary widely. An investigator should be familiar with them and with the types of food with which they are associated.

Food poisoning by bacteria or their products.—Bacteria or their products are responsible for the majority of the outbreaks of food poisoning. Certain of these microörganisms are so prevalent that foods cannot be protected against them. For example, staphylococci are in the throat, on the skin, and in the air and thus have ready access to food.

In bacterial food poisoning the foods involved are usually those in which the causative microörganism can grow. Foods believed to have caused illness are usually thrown into garbage pails before investigations are begun. More often than not, a bacteriological examination has to be made from specimens obtained from waste containers. Obviously, such specimens are subject to bacterial changes, and the interpretation of laboratory data is, of necessity, open to question. Frequently, a particular brand of food is suspected; it is then desirable for an investigator to obtain a sample from the source and, if possible, from the same lot for laboratory examination. In some instances the organism responsible for the food-poisoning outbreak can be isolated from the sample.

People afflicted with food poisoning often erroneously attribute their illness to meat or a meat product which they have eaten. The concept that spoiled meat is a common cause of food poisoning is entirely unfounded and should be discarded. Canned foods are frequently singled out as a cause of illness, without reason. On the other hand, meat and canned foods should not be exempted from consideration and examination along with other food items in any investigation of an outbreak.

Botulism and staphylococcus food poisoning result from eating food in which these organisms have grown and produced their toxins. The symptoms are due entirely to preformed toxins and not to living bacteria.

Botulism gives rise to characteristic symptoms: difficulty in swallowing, double vision, difficulty in speech, labored breathing, and, finally, death from paralysis of the muscles of respiration. These symptoms usually appear within 1–2 days after eating food containing the toxin. Botulism is caused by partaking of improperly processed food in which *Clostridium botulinum* has grown. Since home-canned vegetables are usually involved, it is important to inquire into canning methods.

Staphylococcus food poisoning is characterized by symptoms of nausea, vomiting, diarrhea, and acute prostration arising within $2\frac{1}{2}$–3 hours after eating. Staphylococci may grow rapidly in some foods and produce enterotoxin within a few hours (5–12 or more) when suitable temperatures are provided. Such foods as milk, cured meats, cream-filled bakery goods, etc., are commonly involved.

Salmonella infection of the food-poisoning type is caused by the ingestion of large numbers of salmonella microörganisms. The symptoms are abdominal pain, diarrhea, chills, fever, frequent vomiting, and prostration within 7–72 hours after swallowing the living organisms.

Streptococcus food poisoning is less severe than the other types. The symptoms are nausea, sometimes vomiting, colic-like pains, and diarrhea within 5–12 hours after ingestion of hundreds of millions of these bacteria.

Clostridium perfringens and *Bacillus cereus* are alleged to cause illnesses identical with *Streptococcus faecalis* when they are present in foods in large numbers.

Other types of bacteria have been alleged to cause food poisoning, such as *Escherichia coli* and *Proteus*. The evidence that these microörganisms are causative agents is inconclusive.

OTHER DISEASES TO BE DIFFERENTIATED FROM FOOD POISONING

Epidemics of certain infectious diseases may have some of the properties associated with outbreaks of food poisoning. For example, there are epidemics of acute digestive upsets which are not associated with food or water and are apparently spread by contact infection. These outbreaks do not occur suddenly, and new cases arise over several days' time.

Bacillary dysentery may occur in large outbreaks, but usually secondary cases follow over a period of days or weeks. An outbreak of bacillary dysentery, therefore, lacks the explosive character of an outbreak of food poisoning and may not be related to a specific meal.

Amebic dysentery has a variable period between the swallowing of the cysts of the organism and the onset of symptoms. This period, which may be one of days, months, or years, readily distinguishes it from food poisoning.

The early stages of trichinosis may be confused with food poisoning, since a sudden onset of symptoms may follow a specific meal. The onset is usually about 48 hours after ingestion of the larvae. A history of eating of improperly cooked fresh pork is helpful in making an early diagnosis. The adult worms may also be sought in the stools in the early stages.

REFERENCES

1. HINTZE, K. Geographie und Geschichte der Ernahrung. Leipzig: Georg Thieme, 1934.
2. DONALDSON, R. J. Path. & Bact., **22**:129–51, 1918–19.
3. KERSHAW, G. R. Brit. M. J., **1**:717, 1947.

II *Chemical Poisons in Food*

The literature on chemical poisoning is extensive. In this book only the common types of chemical poisons associated with foods or those which give rise to symptoms confusing them with microbial food poisoning are considered. The reader is referred to standard textbooks of toxicology, especially to W. F. von Oettingen (1), for a more complete coverage of this subject.

Many chemical compounds have been found useful in the production and processing of food. Examples are insecticides, rodenticides, fungicides, and weed control, as well as chemicals which affect the quality of the end-product, such as antioxidants, etc. With the search for new and better chemicals for these purposes, it is important that careful evaluation of the possible health hazards be made for each new compound before its general use is attempted. In the United States House of Representatives, Resolution 323 was passed in the Eighty-first Congress, first session, agreed to on June 20, 1950 (2). This resolution directed a committee headed by James J. Delaney to conduct a full and complete investigation of the following:

1. The nature, extent, and effect of the use of chemicals, compounds, and synthetics in the production, processing, preparation, and packaging of food products to determine the effect of the use of such chemicals, compounds, and synthetics (A) upon the health and welfare of the Nation, and (B) upon the stability and well-being of our agricultural economy;
2. The nature, extent, and effect of the use of pesticides and insecticides with respect to food and food products, particularly the effect of such use of pesticides and insecticides upon the health and welfare of the consumer by reason of toxic residues remaining on such food and food products as a result of such use; and
3. The nature, effect, and extent of the use of chemicals, compounds, and synthetics in the manufacture of fertilizer, particularly the effect of such use of chemicals, compounds, and synthetics upon (A) the condition of the soil as a result of the use of such fertilizer, (B) the quantity and quality of the vegetation growing from such soil, (C) the health of animals consuming such vegetation, (D) the quantity and quality of food produced from such soil, and (E) the public health and welfare generally.

Testimony of representatives of the United States Food and Drug Administration (2) indicated that, of 704 chemicals employed in food use today, only 428 are definitely known to be safe. The Delaney committee felt that the evidence was convincing that chemicals have been utilized in and on the food supply of the nation without adequate testing of their possible long-range injurious effects. The committee pointed out that under existing legislation the government may take no action until after the food has been placed upon the market and injury may have occurred. It was the recommendation of the committee that the Federal Food, Drug, and Cosmetic Act be amended to require that chemicals employed in or on foods be subjected to substantially the same safety requirements as now exist for new drugs and meat products. The investigations of the Delaney committee have stimulated the food industries to investigate chemicals which have contact with food when the chronic toxicity of the chemical is in question.

Chemical poisoning is rare compared to microbial food poisoning. Chemicals such as heavy metals are occasionally taken with suicidal intent or may be maliciously added to foods. A case in point is cited by W. D. McNally. A cook who was never apprehended placed arsenic in soup which was served to 100 people at a banquet given in honor of Archbishop M. in Chicago in 1914. In one quart of the soup 1.227 gm. of arsenic trioxide was found (3).

Chemicals have often been mistaken for articles of food or medicine; for example, sodium fluoride (3) has been mistaken for medicine, baking powder, and starch. As reported by McNally, death occurred in as short a time as 45 minutes in one case and as long as 12 hours in another.

In the literature some food-poisoning outbreaks are mistakenly attributed to chemical poisoning, whereas they probably represent microbial food poisoning. This is illustrated in a letter of Dr. J. C. Geiger (4) to the editor of the *Journal of the American Medical Association* relative to a paper reporting cyanide poisoning from hotel silver polish (5). Geiger points out that final proof of food poisoning should not be accepted without positive laboratory evidence.

A critical review of the literature supports the view that many outbreaks of actual food poisoning have been ascribed to chemical agents in the absence of studies adequate to rule out other causative agents. Thus nickel, aluminum, and copper have popularly been linked with food illnesses—a belief which is not upheld by scientific evidence. Many such outbreaks could be better explained on the basis of bacterial food poisoning, as will be pointed out in a later chapter. On the other hand, several chemicals do actually give rise to food-poisoning symptoms. A list of some of these may be found in Table 1.

Antimony poisoning, which, as mentioned in the Introduction, has resulted from cooking in a poor-quality, gray-enameled cooking utensil, is characterized by vomiting within a few minutes to an hour after ingestion of the chemical. The manufacture of the incriminated product is usually effectively changed when attention is called to such poisoning; but, since unsafe utensils appear on the market from time to time, the possibility of antimony poisoning must be considered.

Arsenic and lead poisoning have been of particular concern among fruit-growers and consumers of sprayed fruit. A group of workers from the Division of Industrial Hygiene at the National Institutes of Health have studied this problem over a period of three years. These workers note that in the fruit-growing district around Wenatchee, Washington, where lead arsenate has been in use for more than a quarter of a century, as much as seven million pounds of this chemical have been applied in one year's time, with results which tend to minimize the danger from spraying fruit with these substances. The people of this area, for the most part, eat raw apples which have not been washed. The following is quoted from two paragraphs in the summary of these investigations (6):

In an effort to investigate even minimal effects of lead arsenate exposure, the population, particularly consumers, was classified by the number of apples they reported eating annually. Separate systems of classification were set up for persons who reported eating commercially-washed apples almost exclusively; for persons who ate unwashed apples almost exclusively; and for persons who ate both washed and unwashed apples. Chemical analyses of unwashed apples of the kind eaten by residents of the district showed that the spray residue lead averaged about 20 times the amount found on apples shipped in interstate commerce.

Clinical and laboratory data for 95 men and 145 women classified as consumers were analyzed in such a way as to trace the effects of the increment in lead and arsenic intake superadded to the usual dietary and atmos-

TABLE 1

CHARACTERISTICS OF GASTROINTESTINAL UPSETS FROM CHEMICAL POISONS

Specific Agent	Food Concerned	Symptoms	Onset of Symptoms
Antimony	Foods cooked in cheap, gray-enameled cooking utensils	Vomiting	Few minutes to an hour
Arsenic	. . . .	Vomiting, diarrhea, painful tenesmus	10 minutes and longer
Barium carbonate	Pastry of tarts	Vomiting, diarrhea, abdominal cramps with tingling sensations in face and neck, followed by loss of tendon reflexes, disordered action of heart, and muscle paralysis	1–2 hours
Cadmium	Acid liquids prepared in cadmium-plated metal utensils	Nausea, vomiting, cramps, and diarrhea	15–30 minutes
Fluoride and sodium fluoride	Sodium fluoride mistaken for baking powder, soda, or flour	Acute poisoning, vomiting, often hemorrhagic, diffuse abdominal pains, and diarrhea occur with great constancy; convulsions, toxic or clonic spasms of certain muscle groups; paresis of certain groups of muscles (eye muscles, facial muscles, hand extensors, and those of lower extremities); hiccough, contraction of pupils, and paresthesia in extremities occasionally present; may be confused with botulism	Few minutes to 2 hours
Lead	. . . .	Abdominal pain, vomiting, and diarrhea in acute cases	30 minutes and longer
Methyl alcohol	Adulterated whiskey	Visual disturbances, weakness, abdominal pain, nausea, vomiting, headache, dizziness, and shortness of breath	Usually 18–48 hours
Methyl chloride	None; leaking mechanical refrigerators	Progressive drowsiness, mental confusion, stupor, weakness, nausea, pain in abdomen, vomiting; convulsions and cyanosis alternating with coma in severe cases; sometimes confused with botulism	Variable
Mercury	. . . .	Astringent metallic taste, salivation, great thirst, vomiting and abdominal pain; watery diarrhea within 2 hours	2–30 minutes after ingesting bichloride of mercury
Nitrates	Water	Cyanosis, vomiting, and diarrhea in infants	Several days
Zinc	Apples cooked in galvanized-iron container	Pain in mouth, throat, and abdomen, followed by diarrhea	. . . .

pheric sources of lead and arsenic. The additional amounts of these elements ingested as lead arsenate on sprayed apples and pears raised the concentration of lead in the blood of male and female consumers to an extent which is more conveniently expressed in micrograms than in milligrams, and also resulted in raising the concentration of lead and arsenic in the urine. For statistical reasons (asymmetrical distribution of urinary lead and urinary arsenic values) the latter two findings cannot be studied as closely as blood lead concentration. These additional amounts of lead arsenate ingested as spray residue were not accompanied by any effects on blood findings (hemoglobin content, erythrocyte count, or reticulocyte percentage) or on the occurrence of any clinical findings, whether considered separately or in associations.

Arsenic poisoning in man occurs most commonly from causes other than adulteration of food—for example, in metallurgical occupations and in patients under treatment for syphilis with arsenical drugs. Lead poisoning is more often an industrial disease than a food poisoning. The extensive use of lead in paints, batteries, gasoline, glazes for pottery, and insecticide sprays makes hazardous the manufacture of these materials. Both arsenic and lead when swallowed in appreciable quantities give rise to acute symptoms of nausea, vomiting, and abdominal pain, which may come on within a period of 10 minutes.

Barium carbonate poisoning involved a total of 85 British soldiers in two outbreaks (7). In the first, 13 men were admitted to a military hospital with acute gastroenteritis. The men became ill 1 hour after their evening meal, which consisted of meat, vegetables, and a marmalade tart. Three sergeants who had not eaten the pastry were not affected. Five soldiers who had only eaten some of the tart also became ill. Before laboratory findings were available for the first outbreak, 71 men in the same unit were taken ill, 2 hours after eating meat, vegetables, and treacle tart. In this second outbreak only the men who ate the tart became ill. A chemical analysis of the pastry revealed large quantities of barium carbonate. At the supply depot a sack containing 4 pounds of barium carbonate to be used for rat poison had been placed, in error, in the flour store, filled with ordinary flour, and issued to the unit.

In a letter of Dr. F. C. Anderson to the editor of the *Journal of the American Medical Association* (8) it is pointed out that boric acid in the amount of 31 gm. to a 2-quart jar of corn has been added by housewives in one area of the United States in canning sweet corn.

The fatal dose of boric acid for an adult is more than 15–20 gm. and for an infant 5–6 gm. This is a dangerous practice and may be more dangerous, since boric acid may be a cumulative poison.

Cadmium poisoning follows the accidental contamination of acid foods and drinks with soluble cadmium compounds. The history of the preparation of the food or drink and the clinical picture are so similar in all outbreaks that the diagnosis is evident to anyone familiar with this type of poisoning (3). The Division of Industrial Hygiene (9) has listed 346 cases of cadmium poisoning reported in the literature from 1858 to 1941; of this number, 287 were due to ingestion, the others being due either to inhalation or to ingestion. However, since this compilation, 300 cases have been reported in a single outbreak (10) in a worker's canteen, which was caused by wine stored in cadmium-lined containers, the cadmium content ranging from 100 to 180 mg. per liter. S. Frant and I. Kleeman (11) describe four outbreaks in New York City from 1937 to 1940. Lemonade, homemade punch, raspberry-gelatin dessert, and tea containing lemon juice were the items of food contaminated with cadmium. The first three of these foods had been placed in ice trays of electric refrigerators for cooling. The ice trays were found to be plated with cadmium. The last item of food was put in a metal pitcher, the inside of which was plated with cadmium. The amount of this element dissolved by these acid foods was 300, 67, 530, and 160 parts per million, respectively. In the case of the smallest amount (67 p.p.m.) symptoms came on within 30 minutes, whereas with the larger amounts of dissolved cadmium, symptoms appeared within 10–15 minutes. The symptoms varied from nausea and abdominal cramps to diarrhea in patients who consumed the largest amounts. Thirteen to 15 p.p.m. of cadmium in "popsicles" (a fruit beverage frozen in a small mold around a wooden stick, which serves as a handle) caused violent nausea in 29 school children; recovery was complete in 5–6 hours. In an Air Force squadron (12) stationed in New Guinea, a mixture of fresh lemons, sugar, and water was prepared only 1 hour before being served to approximately 200 enlisted men. Although the symptoms ranged from mild diarrhea to nausea, vomiting, retching, and abdominal cramps, 27 of the men had to be hospitalized, 2 of whom were in complete shock. The essential features are summarized by Frant and Kleeman as follows:

"The association of immediate food poisoning of groups with the ingestion of an acid liquid prepared in a metal container should cause suspicion, and an immediate investigation for the presence of cadmium-plated utensils should be made."

Fluoride poisoning (13) is due to sodium fluoride, which is often used as an insecticide. It is a white powder, closely resembling baking soda, for which it has been mistaken. Since sodium fluoride is often used to exterminate cockroaches, the package containing this chemical is frequently kept in the kitchen near the food supplies.

H. B. Baldwin (14) describes an outbreak arising from sodium fluoride which was mistakenly substituted for baking powder in making pancakes eaten by 6 or 7 persons. All vomited within 5–15 minutes afterward. In some cases purging occurred, and in one case purging and vomiting continued for a day or more, and the patient also complained of pains in the limbs. One individual who ate 3 or 4 pancakes died within 12 hours. Upon investigation, a box of sodium fluoride roach powder was found by the side of the baking-powder box. In another outbreak described by Baldwin (14), a fairly accurate record of the dosage was obtained. In this outbreak, 26 gm. of fluoride were used instead of baking powder in making 26 wheatcakes for breakfast. If the batter had been equally mixed, each wheatcake should have contained 1 gm. of sodium fluoride. The mother of the family ate 5 cakes, one son 9, another son 1, a daughter 6, and the father 9. The father was seized with cramps almost immediately after eating. Purging commenced early and vomiting within 4 hours. The daughter who ate 6 cakes felt sick when eating the last cake and vomited within 5 or 10 minutes. The mother, who ate 5 cakes, was the most seriously affected. She did not vomit for 5 hours, although diarrhea began within 15 or 20 minutes and continued for several days. These outbreaks illustrate the fact that sodium fluoride may be eaten with food and not discovered by taste. Vomiting and diarrhea are often effective in eliminating much of the poison and make it difficult to determine the fatal dosage for man. Baldwin carried out experiments on himself and found that merely tasting small quantities of sodium fluoride produced a slight feeling of nausea with salivation. As little as 0.25 gm. taken on an empty stomach produced nausea, which was initiated within 2 minutes and reached its greatest intensity in 20 minutes. Vomiting occurred within 2 hours, and nausea continued throughout the following day but disappeared on the second day.

J. C. Geiger (15) reported an outbreak of sodium fluoride poisoning in San Francisco. Poisoning occurred in 21 instances, 3 of which resulted in death. This outbreak was traced to the use of a mixture of sodium bicarbonate and sodium fluoride, sold in bulk as sodium bicarbonate or baking soda.

A large outbreak (16) of sodium fluoride poisoning involving 263 cases with 47 deaths occurred at the Oregon State Hospital at Salem, Oregon. In this outbreak a patient-helper unwittingly mistook roach powder for powdered milk and added approximately 17 pounds of the compound to a 10-gallon mixture of scrambled eggs. The eggs were rejected by many patients because of a salty or soapy taste, while others complained of numbness of the mouth. Nausea, vomiting, and diarrhea occurred abruptly and at times simultaneously. In many instances blood was present in the vomitus and stools. Soon after eating, the patients complained of abdominal burning and cramps. General collapse occurred in severe cases at varying periods of time and was characterized by pallor, weakness, absent or thready pulse, shallow unlabored respiration, weak heart tones, wet cold skin, cyanosis, and equally dilated pupils. Death usually followed. When death was delayed and also in some cases of recovery, there was paralysis of the muscles of deglutition, carpopedal spasm, and spasm of the extremities. Convulsions, abdominal tenderness, and rigidity were absent. In a majority of fatal cases, death occurred 2–4 hours after ingestion of the food, although in a few instances death did not occur for 18–20 hours. In some of the cases, there was local or generalized urticaria, whereas in others there was a thick, mucoid discharge from the mouth and nose.

The cooked eggs contained from 3.2 to 13 per cent sodium fluoride, showing a spotted distribution of the poison. In one patient, who died 15 minutes after ingestion of the eggs, 17.2 gm. of sodium fluoride were present in the stomach. In a patient who died 1 hour after ingestion of the eggs, 3.7 gm. of sodium fluoride were found in the stomach. The stomach of a patient who died 4 hours after eating the eggs was empty, but the liver contained 0.85 gm. of sodium fluoride, and both kidneys held an estimated 0.21 gm. of the poison. In one instance in which death was delayed 18 hours, only 0.18 gm.

of sodium fluoride was found in the stomach. In all cases fluorides were identified by the etch test on glass from the ash in 10-gm. samples of kidney and liver and by the presence of calcium fluoride bands on spectrographic analyses.

At necropsy in sudden deaths, the mucosa of the stomach, duodenum, and first portion of the jejunum was edematous and hyperemic. When death was delayed, petechial hemorrhages of the gastric and duodenal mucosa were observed. The colon was empty except for portions of undigested food, which could be accounted for by the severe diarrhea. There was a general increased wetness and acute congestion of the abdominal viscera, and the liver and kidneys were swollen. The edges of the lungs were ballooned, and occasional interlobar petechial hemorrhages were present. Slight edema and hyperemia were present in the brain.

When eaten by man, 3 gm. of sodium fluoride are sufficient to cause death (17). Fluoride toxicity may result from the formation of an insoluble calcium salt and interference with the action of enzymes and lactic acid metabolism. In 34 fatal cases of poisoning due to fluorine compounds (18), vomiting, diffuse abdominal pains, and diarrhea were common. Convulsions and paresis, often alternating, were a characteristic, but by no means constant, finding. Spasms were confined to certain groups of muscles, especially those of the extremities. Vomiting and diarrhea are often so effective in eliminating fluoride that it may not be recovered by chemical tests of the stomach and contents. Sometimes, however, positive tests are obtained.

Pathologically (17), in sodium fluoride poisoning there is congestion and hemorrhagic infiltration of all the organs, particularly the spleen and lungs. Throughout the pulmonary parenchyma the vessels are so dilated and the vascular channels so congested that blood oozes from the alveoli when the tissue is cut. The liver is yellow, but the edges are sharp and the color uniform. There are no areas of necrosis or acute damage, but cloudy swelling is present. The spleen is enlarged and engorged with erythrocytes. The lymphoid elements are not prominent. The pancreas is macroscopically normal. The kidneys are edematous and moderately swollen. The gastric mucosa is congested and hyperemic, as is the rest of the bowel to a lesser degree. There are small points of hemorrhage in the gastric mucosa, and the stomach contains bloodstained fluid. Symptoms of acute poisoning may occur a few minutes after the ingestion of sodium fluoride, and in fatal cases death supervenes within 6–12 hours or longer.

Sodium fluoride has received considerable study as an anthelmintic for swine (19). It is under consideration as a medicament for the removal of large roundworms, *Ascaris lumbricoides,* from swine when given as 1 per cent of the dry ration for 1 day. This dosage, however, is not without toxic effects on swine, and some animals exhibit symptoms similar to those described for man.

Methyl alcohol poisoning is accompanied, among other symptoms, by abdominal pain, nausea, and vomiting. Like methyl chloride poisoning, it may be confused with botulism, as pointed out by Matheson, Coldwell, and Thatcher (20). Drs. Benton and Calhoun (21) have made an excellent study of a large outbreak in which 320 persons who had ingested adulterated whiskey sought emergency medical care. There were 37 deaths in this group. The adulterated whiskey contained 35 per cent methyl alcohol and 15 per cent ethyl alcohol. Some of these patients had consumed 90 ml. of the alcoholic mixture, and others as much as 750 ml. No correlation was found between the severity of the symptoms and the quantity of methyl alcohol consumed. Visual symptoms studied 18–48 hours after ingestion of the drink included blurred vision, loss of central vision, and complete blindness. There was either no reaction or a sluggish reaction of the pupils to light. Absence of the pupillary light reflex was a sign of poor prognosis for life or eventual restoration of visual acuity. Retinal changes were hyperemia of the optic nerve head and superficial edema of the papilla and surrounding retina, followed by a simple atrophy of the optic nerve. All patients with severe retinal edema had a degree of permanent visual loss. In most patients partial or complete recovery of the initially reduced visual acuity occurred. If visual acuity did not return to normal within 6 days after treatment was begun, it dropped again to a low level.

Acidosis was present in all the severely poisoned patients studied by Benton and Calhoun, and the degree of acidosis paralleled the severity of the general and ocular symptoms. Patients with low blood carbon dioxide values were treated with large doses (25–50 gm.) of sodium bicarbonate intravenously per liter in sterile isotonic glucose, saline solution, or distilled water, which was followed later by oral doses of sodium bicarbonate.

In a discussion of the report of Drs. Benton and Calhoun, Dr. Albert M. Potts (21), of Western Reserve University, points out that methyl alcohol poisoning is not the same in animals as in humans. The lethal dose in grams per kilogram body weight for the rat is ten times higher than for man, and on this basis methyl alcohol is no more toxic for the rat than ethyl alcohol. In Dr. Potts's remarks regarding the mode of action of methyl alcohol in the body, he states: "Subsequent work as yet unpublished shows that the hexokinase system which phosphorylates glucose is the actual site of inhibition."

Methyl chloride poisoning is included in this discussion because the symptoms produced by this type of poisoning have frequently been confused with botulism. Two outbreaks have come to the author's attention in which a clinical diagnosis of botulism had been made by the attending physicians. However, the symptoms in this type of poisoning are sufficiently different to be distinguishable from those of botulism. In methyl chloride poisoning, nausea and vomiting usually initiate the onset of symptoms, whereas in botulism they may or may not be present. The pupils are dilated, and mental confusion and coma are found in methyl chloride poisoning but not in botulism. In Chicago, 29 cases with 10 deaths occurred in 1929 (22). All these cases were due to leaks in kitchenette apartment refrigerators in multiple-unit systems using methyl chloride as the refrigerant. These systems use 100–200 pounds of gas, and a leak in the piping in any one unit may allow great quantities of methyl chloride to escape. Such gaseous poisonings are easily confused with food poisoning if superficially investigated, since many persons in a household may become ill within a short time.

The toxic dosage of methyl chloride for man is not known. W. W. Smith and W. F. von Oettingen (23) present mortality data for dogs and monkeys exposed to methyl chloride in concentrations ranging from 4,000 to 300 p.p.m. on a schedule of 6 hours daily per week. If man is as susceptible to the lethal effects of methyl chloride as dogs and monkeys are, then daily exposure to a concentration of gas of 500 p.p.m. is extremely dangerous even for a period of 2 weeks or less.

In acute mercury poisoning some of the symptoms resemble food poisoning, especially in industrial disease where the pure metal is involved. Similar symptoms also occur when mercuric chloride is mistakenly taken for medicinal purposes or with suicidal intent (see Table 1 for symptoms). However, mercury poisoning is not of importance in food poisoning.

Flour bleached with gaseous nitrogen trichloride (Agene) and fed to dogs was found by Mellanby to cause convulsions (24). Dogs eating a nutritionally adequate diet containing 75 per cent "agenized" white wheat flour (with liver powder and casein and fortified with accessory food substances) developed clinical epilepsy within a week, including typical electroencephalographic patterns, indistinguishable from human idiopathic epilepsy (25). Monkeys showed asynergy, weakness, and tremors, sometimes accompanied by cerebral dysrhythmia. Cats exhibit a marked ataxia, and rats an abnormality of porphyrin metabolism. Mixtures of synthetic amino acids and the individual amino acids, cysteine and cystine, after treatment with Agene, when injected intravenously into dogs on such a diet, produce seizures.

Another group of workers, Newell *et al.* (26), produced running fits in dogs fed high levels of flours bleached with nitrogen trichloride and benzoyl peroxide. Fits did not occur in dogs fed untreated flours or flours treated with benzoyl peroxide, chlorine dioxide, chlorine, nitrogen dioxide, or methyl dichloramine. The toxic factor is associated with the protein of wheat but not with the lipid or carbohydrate. Convulsive seizures have been produced in cats fed agenized flour. It was also found that monkeys fed such flour showed some changes in the electroencephalographic patterns but none of the clinical symptoms associated with running fits. No adverse effect was found on rats, chicks, or guinea pigs. Growth responses of rats and chicks fed nitrogen trichloride–treated whole-wheat flour and unbleached whole-wheat flour were the same. Preliminary studies on 12 human subjects fed agenized wheat products for 2–4 weeks failed to reveal any changes in electroencephalographic patterns, nor were any abnormal clinical symptoms noted.

The Food and Nutrition Board of the National Research Council (27) has taken the position that, in view of the susceptibility of several mammalian species to nitrogen trichloride, there is a definite risk of injury to human beings. Thus nitrogen trichloride is no longer being used as a bleach for flour.

Nitrates in polluted well water, when present in amounts varying from 0.388 gm. of nitrate ion per liter and higher, have been found to cause cyanosis, vomiting, and diarrhea in infants. Severe symptoms occurred in one infant receiving water with a nitrate nitrogen value of 140 p.p.m., which is equivalent to 0.619 gm. of nitrate ion per liter.

Tin poisoning is practically unknown, in spite of the fact that millions of pounds of food packed in tin cans are consumed yearly in this country. Most of the reported outbreaks of food poisoning traced to tin date back many years and, in view of our present knowledge, were probably due to other causes.

The Bureau of Chemistry and Soils of the United States Department of Agriculture carried out feeding experiments in animals and human volunteers with food packed in tin containers. The results, which were negative, apparently have not been published. In a letter concerning these tests, three experiments were detailed, one of which is as follows:

In order to determine the urinary and fecal elimination of tin a human diet squad of four subjects was used. In this experiment the four subjects were placed on a diet shown analytically to be tin free for a preliminary period of 9 days. This was followed by a tin-feeding period of 6 days in which canned pumpkin and canned asparagus were fed. The canned pumpkin was in two separate lots, one of which contained 476 parts per million and the other 383. The canned asparagus contained 361 parts per million of tin. During this tin-feeding period the four subjects ingested a total of 2278 to 2942 milligrams of tin with an average daily ingestion ranging in the four subjects from 426 milligrams to 490 milligrams of tin. During this tin-feeding period the diet was supplemented by such of the tin-free food as the subjects desired. Following the tin period there was a return to the tin-free diet for 10 days which period was divided into three intervals, that is, ending the third, sixth, and tenth days. The urine and feces eliminated by each of the subjects were composited for each of the periods indicated and analyses made for tin. In the urinary samples no tin was found in either the pre-tin, tin, or post-tin periods. In the tin period fecal analyses showed the greatest elimination of tin with diminished amounts in the three samplings of the post-tin period with measurable quantities of tin still present ten days after the tin-feeding period. The elimination of tin through the feces in these human experiments showed 76, 73.8, 91.4, and 91.2 percentages, respectively, for the four subjects. It may be stated that neither during the tin-feeding period nor during the post-tin period did any of the subjects show any evidence of illness or discomfort even after ingesting such abnormally large amounts of tin-containing food [28].

In the next paragraph of the letter this statement is made:

Our own experimental work, involving the ingestion of far larger amounts of tin than any previously reported, and supported by the experimental evidence of other investigators, leads us to the conclusion that tin, in the amounts ordinarily found in canned foods and in the quantity which would be ingested in the ordinary individual diet, is for all practical purposes eliminated and is not productive of harmful effects to the consumer of canned foods.

Luff and Metcalfe (29) describe illnesses in 4 men who opened and ate a can of cherries and a can of meat and also drank some of the cherry juice. In $1\frac{1}{2}$–2 hours they were ill with nausea, vomiting, abdominal cramps, and diarrhea and varying degrees of prostration. The cherries were analyzed, and it was estimated that the doses of malate of tin varied from 4 to 10 grains. Their symptoms are suggestive of staphylococcus food poisoning, which probably arose from enterotoxin in the contaminated canned meat. Subsequent knowledge has failed to show that cherries in tin cans become toxic, while outbreaks of staphylococcus food poisoning from canned meat have been reported.

There is a common concept among the laity that food spoils more quickly when standing in an open tin can than if removed from the can and stored in a separate dish. This is a myth of long standing. Spoilage results from bacteria growing in a food, and, once the food is contaminated, time and suitable temperature will cause spoilage regardless of whether the food is in a tin can or in a glass or porcelain dish. In fact, contamination is less likely to occur if the food is left in the sterile can than if placed in a clean but not sterile dish.

Zinc poisoning in food is so rare that it is usually reported when it is detected. It is associated with acid foods cooked in galvanized-iron kettles. In one outbreak (30) 200 people became ill a few minutes after eating applesauce which was found to contain 1.62 gm. of hydrated zinc sulphate per pound of apples. In another outbreak (31) more or less severe symptoms of poisoning developed in 25 of 42 men who had eaten cooked apples. Chemical tests revealed 83 mg. of zinc in 100 gm. of the food and 17 mg. of zinc in 100 gm. of vomitus. In both outbreaks galvanized-iron kettles had been used for cooking the apples.

Miscellaneous chemicals were in more or less common use many years ago for the preservation of foods (32). Among these were borax or boric acid in milk, meat, butter, oysters, clams, fish, sausage, etc.; formaldehyde in milk; salicylic acid in jams, fruit juices, soda-water syrups, cider, wine, and other sweet preparations; potassium permanganate on the surface of meat to destroy evidence of decomposition; sulphurous acid to preserve and retain the color of fresh meats; and hydrogen peroxide to preserve milk, wine, beer, and fruit juices. Since the passage of the Food and Drug Act of June 30, 1906, the use of these chemicals has been discontinued.

Safety tests for chemicals in foods.—The food technologist is always striving to improve the processing of foods. His objectives have been clearly stated by R. C. Newton (33) as follows:

a) Lower cost of production; this is true whether the food be of plant or animal origin
b) Retard the rate of deterioration from insects, bacteria, enzymes, and chemical change, such as oxidation
c) Lower the cost of processing
d) Improve the method of distribution
e) Improve its convenience to use
f) Improve its palatability with respect to odor, flavor, texture, etc.
g) Retain and improve nutritive quality

In accomplishing these objectives a wide assortment of chemicals such as insecticides, rodenticides, fungicides, herbicides, and others may come in contact with foods during production, processing, and storage. The task of determining whether or not these chemicals are injurious to the health of man is tremendous, expensive, and time-consuming. Obviously, safety testing of chemicals involves the use of experimental animals. The results obtained with man are not always comparable with those for any animal species. For example, as previously mentioned, the rat reacts differently to methyl alcohol than man (21). Dr. Arnold J. Lehman (34) has shown that the dog is more susceptible to the effect of poisons than the rat. Flour bleached with gaseous nitrogen trichloride and fed to dogs caused convulsions (24), whereas no effect was found on rats, chicks, guinea pigs, or man (26). In the case of botulinum toxin, human outbreaks have been traced to types A, B, and E, whereas some animals, such as the mink (35), are resistant to these types but readily develop botulism when fed type C cultures.

From this discussion it is obvious that safety tests should be made on more than one animal species. Since the dietary habits of man and animals differ, it is desirable that a chemical be tested in conjunction with the type of foods in which it would be used. Dr. A. C. Frazer (36, 37, 38) has given an excellent discussion of the pharmacological aspects of chemicals in foods. Among the toxic effects possible are the acute symptoms following the use of tissue irritants. Other chemicals may cause no acute symptoms but effect damage to vital organs. Some chemicals accumulate in the tissues and may concentrate in the kidneys or cumulate. Drugs are usually taken only for a limited time, whereas certain foods are eaten over a lifetime. Therefore, the problem of chronic toxicity is important. Since more information is being developed about carcinogenic drugs, it is important that chemical additives to foods be screened with this possibility in mind. Frazer (36) emphasized the importance of being sure that a chemical additive does not directly interfere with nutritional value. This may result in the following ways: (1) replacing some other dietary constituent of higher nutritional value; for example, substituting high-melting-point fatty-acid esters or polymerized oil for normal fats, which are readily absorbed and have a high caloric value; (2) interfering with the action of alimentary enzymes or with absorption of material of nutritional value; for example, paraffin oil may interfere with absorption of fat-soluble vitamins (39); (3) destroying or altering of essential nutrients by oxidizing or reducing agents; for example, the destruction of vitamins A and E by rancid fats (40, 41).

The screening of an unknown chemical added to, or in contact with, food involving acute and chronic tests in experimental animals is a complicated procedure. In acute toxicity tests the average lethal dose, LD_{50}, should be determined by intraperitoneal injections of graduated dilutions into white mice. Feeding tests with graduated doses should then be made on at least two animal species, such as the white rat and *Macaca mulatta*. Frazer (36) makes this statement regarding the monkey:

Many people have recently suggested monkeys as suitable animals for this type of work. However, precise knowledge of the digestive and absorptive mechanism of monkeys is somewhat scanty; they are essentially herbivorous animals; they are expensive and difficult to maintain; and they frequently suffer from intercurrent diseases which make interpretation of long-term experiments difficult; they hardly seem suitable, therefore, for the investigation of these problems.

This experience of Frazer's has not been that of the author. In the latter's laboratory, *Macaca mulatta* have been used for intestinal surgery and for physiological experiments covering periods of over a year. Care should be exercised by purchasing healthy animals with negative tuberculin tests. Monkeys may be readily fed by stomach tube, and physiologically their intestinal tract is more comparable to man's than is the dog's. Where monkeys cannot be used, dogs are usually the second choice. If the chemical is toxic, as measured by death or tissue damage, or produces any particular effect in 50 per cent of a group of experimental animals as measured in a dietary level expressed in milligrams per kilogram body weight, it is hazardous to consider its use in food at these levels. The arbitrary figure for safety for a chemical in food is often considered as being one hundred times the amount ingested in food and should not give rise to either acute or chronic symptoms of toxicity in the test animals.

Chronic toxicity tests usually cover the life-span of one group of animals, e.g., the rat, and for periods of at least a year in monkeys or dogs. Careful necropsies are made upon all animals sacrificed at test intervals, and the organs are examined histopathologically. Records are kept of organ weights when the animals are sacrificed. In chronic toxicity tests, periodic weights of the animals are taken, as well as food intake. Blood counts and hemoglobin studies are made periodically. Many safety tests are carried through three to five generations in rats.

In chronic toxicity tests, if no toxicity is found in levels of from ten to a hundred times the dosage of chemical encountered in food in the diet, it may be reasonably assumed that the chemical is safe. However, only by extensive trials on man can one be absolutely sure that no harm may arise from the use of the chemical in a food. Observations on man may be made when the product is marketed after safety tests upon animals are completed.

REFERENCES

1. VON OETTINGEN, W. F. Poisoning, p. 524. New York: Paul B. Hoeber, Inc., 1952.
2. Report No. 2356, House of Representatives (82d Cong., 2d sess.), Union Calendar No. 743, June 30, 1952.
3. Toxicology, p. 232. Chicago: Industrial Medicine, 1937.
4. J.A.M.A., **94**:1011, 1930.

5. WILLIAMS, H. J.A.M.A., **94**:627–30, 1930.
6. Pub. Health Bull. 267. Washington: Federal Security Agency, U.S. Pub. Health Service, 1941.
7. MORTON, W. Lancet, **2**:738–39, 1945.
8. J.A.M.A., **157**:484, 1955.
9. Pub. Health Rep., **57**:601–12, 1942.
10. MONNET, R., and SABON, F. Presse méd., **54**:677, 1946.
11. FRANT, SAMUEL, and KLEEMAN, IRVING. J.A.M.A., **117**:86–89, 1941.
12. GARBER, J. S. Bull. U.S. Army M. Dept., **5**:349–50, 1946.
13. GREENWOOD, D. A. Physiol. Rev., **20**:582–616, 1940.
14. BALDWIN, HERBERT B. J. Am. Chem. Soc., **21**:517–21, 1899.
15. GEIGER, J. C. California & West. Med., **44**:81–83, 1936.
16. LIDBECK, WILLIAM L., HILL, IRVIN B., and BEEMAN, JOSEPH A. J.A.M.A., **121**:826–27, 1943.
17. CARR, JESSE L. California & West. Med., **44**:83–86, 1936.
18. ROHOLM, KAJ. Fluorine intoxication, pp. 26–27. London: Lewis & Co., 1937.
19. HABERMANN, R. T., ENZIE, F. D., and FOSTER, A. O. Am. J. Vet. Res., **6**:131–44, 1945.
    ENZIE, F. D., HABERMANN, R. T., and FOSTER, A. O. J. Am. Vet. M. A., **107**:57–66, 1945.
    ALLEN, REX W. North Am. Vet., **26**:661–64, 1945.
    ALLEN, REX W., and JONES, LLOYD DIEHL. North Am. Vet., **27**:358–60, 1946.
20. MATHESON, B. H., COLDWELL, B., and THATCHER, F. S. Canad. M. A. J., **72**:139, 1955.
21. BENTON, CURTIS D., JR., and CALHOUN, F. PHINIZY, JR. Tr. Am. Acad. Ophth., **56**:875–85, 1952.
22. KEGEL, ARNOLD H., McNALLY, WILLIAM D., and POPE, ALTON S. J.A.M.A., **93**:353–58, 1929.
23. SMITH, W. W., and VON OETTINGEN, W. F. J. Indust. Hyg. & Toxicol., **29**:47–52, 1947.
24. MELLANBY, E. Brit. M. J., **2**:885–87, 1946.
25. SILVER, MAURICE L., JOHNSON, ROBERT E., KARK, ROBERT M., KLEIN, J. RAYMOND, MONAHAN, ELMER P., and ZEVIN, SOLOMON S. J.A.M.A., **135**:757–60, 1947.
26. NEWELL, G. W., ERICKSON, T. C., GILSON, W. E., GERSHOFF, S. N., and ELVEHJEM, C. A. J.A.M.A., **135**:760–63, 1947.
27. FOOD AND NUTRITION BOARD OF THE NATIONAL RESEARCH COUNCIL. J.A.M.A., **135**:769–70, 1947.
28. Letter dated October 19, 1929, to Mr. F. E. Gorrell, of the National Canners Association, from Henry G. Knight, chief of Bureau of Chemistry and Soils, United States Department of Agriculture.
29. LUFF, ARTHUR P., and METCALFE, G. H. Brit. M. J., **1**:833–34, 1890.
30. Brit. M. J., **1**:201, 1923.
31. DORNICKX, C. G. J. Nederl. tijdschr. geneesk., **82**:4185–4294, 1938; abstr., J.A.M.A., **111**:1887, 1938.
32. ROSENAU, M. J. Prevent. Med. & Hyg., 6th ed., pp. 739–47, 1935.
33. NEWTON, R. C. The Canner, **114**:14, 1952.

34. Lehman, Arnold J. Association of Food and Drug Officials of the United States, Bull. 16, pp. 47–53, 1952.
35. Wagenaar, R. O., Dack, G. M., and Mayer, D. P. Am. J. Vet. Res., **14**:479–83, 1953.
36. Frazer, A. C. J. Sc. Food & Agriculture, **2**:1–7, 1951.
37. ———. Proc. Roy. Soc. Med., **45**:37–40, 1952.
38. ———. Endeavour, Vol. **12**, January, 1953.
39. Alvarez, W. C. Gastroenterology, **9**:315, 1947.
40. Mattill, H. A. J.A.M.A., **110**:1831, 1938.
41. Whipple, D. J. Pediat., **8**:734, 1936.

III *Poisonous Plants and Animals*

Snakeroot, poisonous mushrooms, water hemlock, rhubarb leaves, and such plants give rise to gastrointestinal symptoms. Other plants and animals—shellfish, certain fish, fava beans, and a parasitic fungus of rye—elicit various types of poisoning without gastrointestinal upsets. Data relevant to the poisoning associated with the more important of these forms may be found in Table 2 (pp. 32 and 33). Other plant or animal poisonings which are rare or not well established are not discussed.

SHELLFISH POISONING

Shellfish have commonly been associated with gastrointestinal illness and typhoid fever. An excellent study was reported by Dr. H. Timbrell Bulstrode (1), who called attention to the hazards of contamination of shellfish with sewage. He reported 10 outbreaks dating from 1827 to 1890 attributed to poisoning by mussels. The following statement is made regarding the first of these: "In 1827 some thirty persons were severely affected—in two cases fatally—after eating mussels taken from the dock gates at Leith, and a cat and dog to which some of the mussels were given were similarly affected." Paralysis of the voluntary muscles and absolute unconsciousness were described for one of 3 patients in an outbreak in 1888.

Meyer (2) has called attention to the many outbreaks of typhoid fever caused by contaminated mussels and has reviewed the literature on shellfish poisoning, which is an intoxication unrelated to infection with enteric microörganisms. He also points to the worldwide distribution of shellfish poisoning. The intoxication is characterized by variable gastrointestinal symptoms in man, which is secondary to the paresthesias and paralysis that may appear within 10 minutes of the ingestion of the offending shellfish or shellfish broth. Tingling and numbness of the lips are followed by prickly feelings in the fingertips. Ataxia and giddiness, staggering, and drowsiness are frequently present. Mental symptoms are variable;

TABLE 2

CHARACTERISTIC SYMPTOMS DUE TO POISONOUS PLANTS OR ANIMALS

Disease	Specific Agent	Food Concerned	Symptoms	Onset of Symptoms
Shellfish poisoning	Plankton (*Gonyaulax*), food of mussels	Mussels	Respiratory paralysis; milder symptoms consist of trembling about lips to complete loss of power in the muscles of extremities and neck	5–30 minutes and longer
Asari and oyster poisoning	Unknown	Asari and oysters	Anorexia, abdominal pain, nausea, vomiting, constipation, and headache	24 hours to 7 days
	1. Tetraodontoxin in liver and ovaries	"Blowfish," *fugu*, globefish, *toado*, puffer	Numbness and tingling of lips, tongue, fingers, and toes; loss of taste, respiratory paralysis in fatal cases; nausea, vomiting, abdominal pain, and ataxia usually present	30 minutes to several hours
	2. Ciguatera toxin	Snapper	Epigastric pain, numbness in limbs, tingling about face, giddiness, watery stools, slow pulse, contracted pupils; tingling sensation over whole body, especially lips and fingers; ataxia, myalgia, muscular weakness	Few minutes to 30 hours
Fish poisoning (ichthyosarcotoxism)	3. Gymnothorax toxin	Gymnothorax Moray eel (*Gymnothorax buroensis* [Bleeker]), *G. flavimarginatus* (Ruppell), *G. javanicus* (Bleeker), *G. meleagris* (Shaw and Nodder), *G. petelli* (Bleeker), *G. pictus* (Ahl), *G. undulatus* (lacepede)	Tingling and numb sensation about the lips, vomiting, coma, perspiration, nausea, aphonia, foaming at mouth, convulsions, respiratory paralysis	20 minutes to 7–8 hours
	4. Scombroid toxin	Fish of genera *Euthynnus* and *Katsuwonus*	Nausea, vomiting, redness and flushing of face, engorgement of soft tissues of eyes, swelling and cyanosis of lips, tongue, and gums, giant urticaria, severe itching, headache, and respiratory distress	Within a few minutes
	5. Elasmobranch toxin	Shark's liver; *Prionace glauca* (Linnaeus), *Mustelus canis* (Mitchill), *Squatina dumeril* (Lesueur), and *Somniosus microcephalus* (Bloch and Schneider)	Generalized malaise, joint aches, headache, nausea, vomiting, diarrhea, extreme fatigue, severe ataxia, violent pruritus, desquamation, spasmodic contraction of eyelids, respiratory distress, cold sweats, delirium, coma, and death in many cases	Unknown
	6. Fresh-water fish poison	Roe or gonads of minnows of family Cyprinidae European barbel, *Barbus barbus*	Headache, fever, dizziness, vomiting, colic and diarrhea, anuria, pallor, and prostration	Within a few minutes to 6 hours

32

TABLE 2—*Continued*

Disease	Specific Agent	Food Concerned	Symptoms	Onset of Symptoms
Akee poisoning	Seeds and arils of un-ripe akee	Akee nuts	Violent vomiting	2–3 hours
Favism	Bean, *Vicia fava*, or inhalation of pollen from blossoming plant	Bean, *Vicia fava*	Acute febrile anemia, with jaundice, hematuria, and hemoglobinuria	1 hour after eating beans in 1 case
Snakeroot poisoning	Trematol from snakeroot (*Eupatorium urticaefolium*)	Milk from cows pastured on snakeroot	Weakness or prostration, pernicious vomiting, severe constipation, and epigastric pain; temperature normal	Variable period; after repeated use of milk from cows pastured in area where snakeroot is present
Mushroom poisoning	Phalloidine and other alkaloids	Poisonous mushrooms (*Amanita phalloides* and other species)	Hypoglycemia and convulsions; severe abdominal pain, intense thirst, nausea, retching, vomiting, and profuse watery evacuations sometimes containing blood and mucus	6–15 hours
Ergotism	Parasitic fungus of rye (*Claviceps purpurea*)	Rye meal or bread	Gangrenous, involves limbs, especially fingers and toes, occasionally ears and nose; convulsions, depression, weakness and drowsiness, headache, giddiness, painful cramps in limbs, and itching of skin	Gradually, after several meals
Water-hemlock poisoning	Cicutoxin or resin from water hemlock (*Cicuta maculata*)	Leaves and roots of water hemlock	Nausea, vomiting, and convulsions	1–2 hours
Poison honey	Rhododendron (*Andromeda*) eaten by bees	Honey	Nausea, vomiting, diarrhea, dizziness, headache, temporary blindness, fainting, fever, complete unconsciousness	Unknown
Potato poisoning	Solanine (Glucoalkaloid)	Potatoes	Not toxic to man unless eaten in quantity of 17.6 lb. at one time	. . . .
Rhubarb poisoning	Oxalic acid (in greens)	Rhubarb greens	Cramplike pains, failure of blood to clot, possibly death	2–12 hours
Tung-nut poisoning	Tung seeds	Tung-nut tree (*Aleurites fordii*)	Nausea, vomiting, diarrhea, and abdominal cramps	30 minutes

33

there may be dryness and gripping sensations of the throat and incoherence of speech. If the patient survives for 12 hours, the prognosis is good. In some cases a complete aphasia is observed. Where death occurs in severe cases, it is due to respiratory failure. No significant findings have been reported upon necropsy.

In July, 1927, in San Francisco and vicinity, approximately 102 cases of mussel poisoning occurred suddenly. These outbreaks attracted attention in the daily press and gave rise to an investigation by the California State Department of Health and the State Fish and Game Commission. Of the 102 people in the outbreak, 56 were men (twenty-four to sixty-five years of age), 8 boys (two to twelve years of age), 34 women (twenty to sixty years of age), and 4 girls (thirteen to fifteen years of age). Those ill had eaten steamed, cooked, or raw mussels of a Pacific Coast variety (*Mytilus californianus*), freshly gathered in various localities within a radius of 45 miles south and 50 miles north of the Golden Gate. Meyer and others (3) tabulated 20 outbreaks of mussel poisoning in the world, beginning with one reported in 1793. Since then, approximately 244 people have been poisoned, and 38 have died.

From 1927 to 1947 the records for the Pacific Coast (4) show 409 cases of mussel and clam poisoning and 35 deaths. Most cases occurred along the central California coast, with a sprinkling of severe outbreaks from Juneau, Alaska, to southern California and the Gulf of California, Mexico. All cases appeared between May 15 and October 26.

Shellfish poisoning has been reported in certain shellfish in Nova Scotia (5). In July, 1936, Dr. P. S. Campbell, chief health officer of Nova Scotia, reported to the Department of Pensions and National Health the occurrence of a few cases of severe illness in Digby County following the consumption of mussels. Two of the cases were fatal. The poison was found to be similar to that reported in California. Two species of mussels were found to be toxic, i.e., *Mytilus edulis* and *Modiola modiolus*.

In a survey (6) of commercially important shellfish areas of this region, paralytic shellfish poison has been found in shellfish only from the Bay of Fundy area in the late summer and early fall. In August, 1945, in New Brunswick, 21 cases of poisoning were recorded. All these cases resulted from eating clams whose toxicities were above 6,000 mouse units (MU).[1] The mean consumption of poison required to produce mild, severe, and extreme symptoms of poisoning in susceptible persons was found to be about 7,000, 16,000, and 32,000 MU, respectively.

In 1946 (2) an epidemiological investigation of an outbreak of mussel poisoning was made, whereby information concerning the toxicity of mussels eaten and the exact number of mussels which each of 3 people ate was established. A man consuming 42,000 MU died in less than 4 hours. A woman, consuming 22,000 MU, became seriously ill but recovered after being placed in a respirator for $4\frac{1}{2}$ hours. A second man, who had eaten mussels containing 17,000 MU, had mild symptoms but recovered. The smallest dose to give rise to symptoms was estimated to be 15,000 MU. Food and Drug Administration regulations on commercial canned shellfish do not permit more than 1,200 MU per 100 gm. of shellfish meat.

A history of a typical case, taken from Meyer and others (3) (case 2), follows:

A middle-aged well-built man called at the laboratory. He had an ataxic gait but spoke distinctly and stated that he had been poisoned by eating mussels. On Sunday, July 17, at 1:00 P.M. during low tide he gathered mussels which were submerged at a place approximately three miles west of Pescadero. No sewage discharges into the sea within twenty miles. Late in the afternoon the carefully washed shell-fish were steamed for about 12 or 15 minutes. The hot and thoroughly cooked mollusks tasted good and he ate about 2 quarts (three dozen small size) and his wife about 6 small mussels during the evening meal. About 15 minutes after eating he felt nauseated but could not vomit. He felt drowsy, went to bed, and had a restless sleep continually interrupted by dreams. Although he did not feel well in the morning he went to his business. About 10:30 A.M. he noticed a general numbness around his lips, chin and cheeks[2] and particularly in the thumb of the left hand. These symptoms still persisted during his examination on July 18. The reflexes were present and active, the pupils reacted to light and were dilated. The temperature was 98.4° F. The numbness gradually disappeared during the afternoon. The broth (0.5 cc.) of the steamed mussels killed a mouse within 3 minutes.

During the meal the patient fed several mussels to 3 half grown kittens and one cat, and two mollusks to a police dog. The dog vomited within 20

1. The mouse unit (MU), or average lethal dose, has been defined (H. Sommer and K. F. Meyer, Arch. Path., 24:560–98, 1937) as that amount of mussel poison which, when dissolved in 1.0 ml. of water and injected intraperitoneally into a 20-gm. white mouse, will cause death in 15 minutes.

2. The symptoms of numbness around the lips, chin, and cheeks, of which this man complained, have in other cases appeared in less than an hour.

minutes but was not otherwise affected. The 3 kittens died during the night at the same place where the food had been offered in the evening. The cat showed a complete posterior paralysis 18 hours after eating mussels, but recovered.

During the years which followed the 1927 outbreak in California, work on this problem was continued at the George Williams Hooper Foundation at the University of California. Many theories were advanced to explain the occurrence of the poison in shellfish. The hypothesis that the toxic agent is an organism pathogenic for mussels or the assumption that the toxicity is due to an actual disease has not been supported by fact. Many theories were abandoned as it became more apparent that the agent responsible for the toxicity is contained in the ocean water and approaches the shellfish beds more or less periodically from offshore. The search for the causative factor narrowed down to a dissolved or particulate substance in the water which the mussels were absorbing. The food of the shellfish, i.e., the diatoms and dinoflagellates, was next considered. The poison has been detected in and extracted from plankton (7). Samples of plankton collected frequently during the summer months of 1935 yielded amounts of poison roughly proportional to the numbers of the dinoflagellate, *Gonyaulax catenella*, present. On the average, 3,000 of these organisms yielded 1 MU of poison. The dinoflagellate, *G. catenella* (4, 8), is a free-swimming organism of dark-orange or greenish-brown color, which multiplies by the formation of chains of two, four, or even eight individuals and lives like a true plant cell by photosynthesis. It may multiply to such an extent that the water presents a deep rust-red color, so-called "red water," which may be seen for miles in the daytime and is a beautiful, luminescent spectacle at night.

A method has been devised for detecting and quantitatively estimating the poison in shellfish. It consists in measuring amounts of alcohol-soluble extracts of the livers of the shellfish by injecting mice intraperitoneally.

The poison.—This poison (7) is one of the strongest known. It belongs to the class of alkaloids, such as strychnine, muscarine, and aconitine. It is readily soluble in water and alcohol but insoluble in ether and chloroform. The stability of the poison (9) in aqueous solution decreases with an increase in pH and temperature. The mussel poison has been concentrated by the use of ion exchange on a synthetic zeolite (barium or sodium Decalso). With this method, it was possible to obtain a 50–70 per cent yield of the poison, with a toxicity of 70–140 MU/mg, an increase in potency of eighteen fold. The fatal dose for man is probably a few milligrams by mouth.

A procedure (10) has been developed for the chromatographic fractionation of mussel poison concentrates on active carbon. The adsorption behavior of mussel poison on active carbon was found to vary widely with different anions. By chromatography on Norit A of mussel poison concentrates obtained from ion exchange on Decalso, it was possible to obtain a yield of 30–50 per cent of twenty fold enriched material with a toxicity greater than 1.00 MU/μgm. The chromatography of partially decolorized, defatted, crude mussel poison extracts on Norit A was found to yield 30–50 per cent of seventy-five fold enriched material.

Riegel *et al.* (11) have precipitated mussel poison as the rufianate, helianthate, and reineckate without losing its pharmacological activity. Mussel poison sulphate has been prepared. Large-scale purification of mussel poison has been accomplished by crystallization of the helianthate. Betaine, choline, homarine, taurine, and tyrosine have been isolated and identified in liver extracts from poison mussels. Choline and homarine, both quaternary bases, are closely associated with the poison through preliminary steps in purification. An additional base has been detected by its characteristic ultraviolet absorption spectrum but has not been identified.

A large-scale collection of marine plankton (11) rich in *G. catenella* was made by passing water containing large numbers of the plankton through supercentrifuges. Concentration by chromatography on acid-washed Norit A furnished a fraction of poison with a toxicity of 1.65 MU/μgm. The chemical structure of the toxic principle is still to be determined (12).

Sampling.—Since the variation in toxicity of mussels in a given bed is not large, the standard sample is limited to a few mussels, whose length, weight, and volume are considered. Volume seems to be a better criterion than weight, since it is not affected by shell water as the weight is. It is measured by immersing the mussels in tap water in a graduated cylinder. The shells of live animals under such conditions are always tightly closed, and no error is likely to occur from imbibition of water. Sommer and Meyer (4) use the following procedure for sampling: generally, three or four mussels are selected, the combined length of which measures 10 inches (25 cm.). The volume is determined and the results of the test expressed in units of poison per 100 cc. of whole mussel.

Test for poison in clams or mussels (13).—The livers of the mussels or the livers plus syphons of the clams are used. Ten ml. of 0.1 N hydrochloric acid per shellfish are customarily employed for extraction. The tissue is ground with the dilute acid, and the mixture is boiled gently for approximately 5 minutes. After centrifugation or filtration, the liquid is ready for injection. The results are expressed in mouse units per 50 gm. of mussel or per clam; the poison content may vary from less than 10 to over 10,000 MU per shellfish.

In the case of canned or fresh clams the following standard test has been widely adopted: 100 gm. of ground clam meats are extracted with 100 ml. of hydrochloric acid 0.1–0.2 N, and the extract is prepared as above. (The strength of the acid depends on the species of clam, 0.1 N for Little Neck clams, 0.05–0.2 N for Washington clams.) The mixture should at all times react acid to Congo paper. The results are expressed in mouse units per 100 gm. of clam meats.

Sommer and Meyer analyzed mussels from numerous places between central California and southern Oregon. Besides the shellfish mentioned, seven of the common varieties of edible clams were found to contain the poison in smaller amounts. Poisonous mussels were found to be indistinguishable from normal ones, except by the animal test. Mussels subjected to various conditions in the laboratory have never shown an increase in toxicity; they usually show detoxification, the rate of which has been determined. The poison was also demonstrated, during the poison season, in the residue of filtered sea water.

No specific treatment has been found for this disease. The treatment of cases with apomorphine to produce vomiting has been found more effective than gastric lavage. Digitalis and alcohol are contraindicated.

Asari and oyster poisoning in Japan.—Akiba and Hattori (14) reported that in March, 1942, in the district along Lake Hamana, 324 cases of poisoning occurred and, of this number, 114 (34 per cent) died. Symptoms appeared 1–7 days following the eating of a large number of asari (*Venerupis semidecussata*). In March of the following year (1943) an essentially identical type of poisoning followed the eating of oysters (*Ostrea gigas*). In March, 1949, an identical type of poisoning involving 93 persons, with 6 (6.5 per cent) deaths, occurred in the same district from eating asari or oysters. In another district in Japan 2 outbreaks with the same symptoms occurred, the one in 1889 and the other in 1941.

The symptoms developed 24–48 hours after consumption of the toxic bivalves and were characterized by anorexia, abdominal pain, nausea, vomiting, constipation, and headache. Early after symptoms developed, petechiae appeared on the chest, neck, and upper parts of the arms and legs. The temperature was usually normal. Blood was often observed in the vomitus, and bleeding occurred from the mucous membrane of the nose, gingiva, and uterus. In fatal cases excitability was followed by delirium. Laboratory examination revealed leukocytosis, lengthening of blood coagulation time, and disturbance of liver function.

Necropsy findings showed an acute yellow atrophy of the liver and a hemorrhagic diathesis. Histologically, there was a fatty degeneration of the liver cells.

The Lake Hamana area, where the toxic asari and oysters were found, was near the mouth of the lake through which the tide flows in and out. Asari and oysters gathered in other places relatively distant from the district were nontoxic. Persons eating only a few (10–15) bivalves were not made ill, whereas those eating 40–60 or more (150–250 gm. tissue) were. The tissues from 100 shells were ingested in the fatal cases.

The toxic principle was most abundant in the livers of the bivalves and could readily be precipitated by absolute alcohol. Akiba and Hattori (14) considered it different from mussel poisoning, previously described in America, because it was destroyed by the hydrochloric acid used to acidulate the methyl alcohol employed for extraction. The poison (pH 5.4) was not destroyed by boiling for 3 hours or heating for 1 hour at 109° C., but from 50 to 85 per cent was destroyed by heating for 30–60 minutes at 115°–119° C. Dogs, cats, rabbits, and mice have been intoxicated by oral, intravenous, intraperitoneal, or subcutaneous injection of the poison.

There was no relationship between the spawning period of the bivalves and their toxicity. Nontoxic asari became toxic 10 days after transplantation in waters containing the toxic bivalves. Furthermore, the toxicity of highly poisonous oysters fell markedly shortly after transplantation to safe districts. Akiba (15) found the plankton, *Rhizosolenia hebetate,* to be the predominating one during the period of greatest toxicity. He was unable to extract the poison from the plankton, and shellfish cultivated in pots with *R. hebetate* failed to develop toxin. He was unable to find *Gonyaulax catenella* in these waters.

FISH POISONING (ICHTHYOSARCOTOXISM)

The intoxication resulting from the ingestion of the flesh of poisonous fish has been named "ichthyosarcotoxism" (from the Greek *ichthyos,* "a fish"; *sarkos,* "flesh"; *toxikon,* "poison") by one of the foremost students of fish poisoning, Dr. Bruce W. Halstead (16). Halstead has completed a survey of nearly fifteen hundred publications on the subject of poisonous and venomous marine animals from all parts of the world, and he found that, during the last 200 years, about 518 species of fish involving 95 families have been incriminated as poisonous. Thirty-eight were of commercial importance.

Since the poisons associated with the various types of fish poisoning have not been characterized chemically and since the pharmacology of the various types of fish poisons has not been thoroughly studied, any groupings of ichthyosarcotoxism must be regarded as tentative. Dr. Halstead believes that there are six distinctly different clinical entities comprising ichthyosarcotoxism, involving the following groups of fish: (1) tetraodon (puffer, *fugu,* globefish, *toado,* etc.), (2) ciguatera, (3) gymnothorax, (4) scombroid, (5) elasmobranch, and (6) fresh-water fish.

Tetraodon (puffer) poisoning.—Professor Ichiro Tokuyama (17), from the Medical School at Kyushu University in Fukuoka, Kyushu, Japan, has detailed some information about poisoning which occurs in Japan from eating the blowfish (*fugu*). There are several of these species, most of which are not edible. An edible type is called by the Japanese *Mafugu.* The poison is in the visceral organs. In some prefectures in Japan cooks must have a license to cook and serve this fish to the public, while in others the sale of visceral organs is prohibited. There are several species of the Tetraodontes which do not possess the toxin. However, the most choice edible species harbor the toxin, which is located in the liver and ovaries. Tetraodontoxin is a highly toxic neurotoxin which withstands boiling. Its exact chemical nature is unknown. The organs from a single fish, when eaten, may be lethal to man.

Loss of taste is one of the first symptoms to appear, and eventually in fatal cases respiratory paralysis occurs. The mild toxic symptoms are said to resemble alcoholic intoxication, and the toxic organs are ingested in small amounts by some people to attain that effect. No antidote for the poisoning has been found, and severe cases are almost always fatal. In small doses the toxin has been used for the relief of neuralgic pain.

Halstead and Bunker (18) tested tissue extracts from samples of musculature, liver, gonads, and intestines of four common Japanese puffers, both before and after a canning process to determine the heat lability of the toxin. Canning was carried out according to commercial practice, and the cases were heated in a steam retort under a pressure of 12.5 pounds per square inch at 116.°6 C. for 75 minutes. The toxin was partially, but not completely, destroyed by this treatment. Extracts from the liver and gonads of *Sphoeroides* var. *radiatus* were only slightly affected by the heating process.

Ciguatera.—The term "ciguatera" came from the early Spanish settlers of Cuba, who used it in connection with neurological and gastrointestinal disturbances resulting from eating the marine snail, *Turbo pica,* otherwise known as *cigua.* Ciguatera now generally refers to ichthyosarcotoxism. Robert L. Gilman (19) has described fish poisoning in the Puerto Rico–Virgin Islands area which was probably ciguatera. Ross (20) reported an outbreak of fish poisoning in the Fanning Islands in the central Pacific. From February, 1946, to April 5, 1947, there were 95 cases of fish poisoning at Fanning among a population of 224 people on the island. In cooking fish, the natives wrap the whole fish in pandanus or palm leaves and place them over burning coconut husks. On September 19, 1946, at 3:00 P.M., a snapper (*makura*), weighing about 5 pounds, was caught from an American Army ship. The fish was cleaned and put on ice, and the flesh was fried at 4:00 P.M. At 5:00 P.M. it was eaten by 4 members of the crew and 4 Chinese laborers. All 8 people were ill about 4 and 5 hours after eating the fish. The symptoms were epigastric pain, numbness in limbs, tingling around the face, and giddiness. Two patients had severe vomiting, but the rest vomited only once. All had watery stools about 2 hours after the onset of illness. The next morning they had slow pulses (30–40 per minute), contracted pupils, and a sensation of tingling over the whole body, especially about the lips and fingertips, and noticed a feeling of coldness when the hands or feet were immersed in water at room temperature. This effect was apparent in 6–8 hours after the onset in 5 patients and in 20–24 hours in 3 patients.

Cats, dogs, and domestic ducks fed poisonous fish experimentally or accidentally developed within 8–12 hours an ascending paralysis, which lasted from 3 to 5 days. Of 55 cases studied due to ingesting 10 different kinds of poisonous fish, 19 patients had eaten the whole fish, and 36 had eaten only the flesh.

Fish poisoning has been studied by the Japanese, and several series of their papers have been translated into English by W. G. Van Campen (21). Yoshio Hiyama, one author in the group, studied poisonous fish in the Marianas and Marshall Islands and described 45 toxic species. He mentions that not all 45 species when eaten give rise to identical symptoms, and he does not assume that the same toxic agent is involved. In reading numerous descriptions of outbreaks of fish poisoning, however, there appears to be a remarkable similarity in symptoms, as can be noted in outbreaks detailed in this chapter. The poison is said to be readily extracted in water or alcohol. The Japanese fishermen of Saipan, according to Takashi Yasukawa (21), remove the poison from mildly toxic species in the following manner:

> They split open the belly and remove the viscera and then soak the fish overnight in ice water. The next day they pound the flesh up fine, wash it in water several times, add wheat flour and make it into fishcake or fish pudding for sale. It is said that this method has been employed for years without any cases of poisoning resulting. It is not known at present whether this is due to the washing away of the blood or whether the poison is extracted from muscle tissues, but it is reported here as a presumably effective method.

Gymnothorax (Moray eel) poisoning.—Khlentzos (22) describes an outbreak among Filipino civilians at Saipan, who on May 8,

1949, at 11:00 A.M. caught an eel by spearing the tail and then hooking the neck. The eel, *Gymnothorax flavimarginatus,* measured about 6 feet long and 1 foot thick. At camp the eel was cleaned and cut into steaks, and half, together with the head, was placed into a large pot of water and boiled, with black pepper, vinegar, and salt added. After cooking for 30 minutes, one-quarter of a slice was consumed by each of 57 Filipinos at 7:00 P.M. A scratchy sensation in the mouth and throat occurred at the time the fish was eaten. About 20 minutes later, tingling and numb sensations were described about the lips. Approximately 30 minutes after eating, some of the feasters were unable to talk, and all 57 went to the dispensary on Saipan, where each had a gastric lavage. One and a half hours after eating the eel, some men experienced syncope and fell. During their stay at the Saipan Station Hospital, about 50 vomited. After 4 hours at the dispensary, all were sent back to their camp. Twenty-four to 48 hours later these patients experienced numbness of their mouths, and some were unable to talk. Two dogs fed the cooked eel on the evening of May 8 were dead the next morning.

Seventeen of the 57 men were hospitalized. Of these 17 patients, 11 were admitted in coma, and 3 of the remaining 6 became comatose after a few hours. Treatment was symptomatic, the symptoms causing a major nursing problem. Thirteen of the 17 patients, upon admission to the hospital, showed an absence of thoracic respiration, with prominent abdominal breathing; 4–7 days were required for thoracic respiration to be restored. Tonic and clonic convulsions were seen in a number of patients. One death occurred after 14 days and one after 20 days. Perspiration was profuse in 12 patients during the first week, with as much as 500–1,000 ml. being produced in a matter of minutes. Eight patients had trismus. The duration of unconsciousness varied from 2 to 10 days. Areflexia continued from 30 to 60 days.

Scombroid poisoning (Tjakalang poisoning).—Members of the genera *Euthynnus* and *Katsuwonus* are the most common offenders, but other types of scombroid fish, such as tuna, mackerel, bonito, albacore, and skipjack, have been involved (23). In rare instances these fish may produce symptoms typical of the ciguatera type of fish poisoning. The symptoms generally develop within a few minutes after ingesting the fish and consist of nausea, vomiting, redness and flushing of the face, engorgement of the soft tissues of the eyes, swelling and cyanosis of the lips, tongue, and gums, giant urticaria, severe itching, headache, and respiratory distress. The victim usually recovers within 8–12 hours. This is the only form of ichthyosarcotoxism associated with inadequate refrigeration or freshness of the fish. The few bacteriological analyses of the fish flesh which have been made have not revealed the cause. Van Veen and Latuasan (24) have described this poisoning in the Dutch East Indies, where a variety of bonito (*E. pelamis* L.; skipjack; striped tuna) was involved.

Elasmobranch poisoning (23).—Several species of sharks have been incriminated, but their identification is questionable. Species which appear certain are *Prionace glauca* (Linnaeus), the great blue shark; *Mustelus canis* (Mitchill), the smooth dogfish; *Squatina dumeril* (Lesueur), the angel shark; and *Somniosus microcephalus* (Bloch and Schneider), the Greenland shark. The usual symptoms follow eating of the liver and are characterized by generalized malaise, joint aches, headaches, nausea, vomiting, diarrhea, extreme fatigue, severe ataxia, violent pruritus, desquamation, spasmodic contraction of the eyelids, respiratory distress, cold sweats, delirium, coma, and death. Recoveries have occurred in many cases. There is no known treatment, and the relationship, if any, of elasmobranch poisoning to ciguatera poisoning is not understood.

Fresh-water fish poisoning.—A number of species of the family Cyprinidae or the fresh-water minnows, such as the European barbel, *Barbus barbus* (Linnaeus), have been incriminated. Symptoms develop in from a few minutes up to 6 hours following the eating of the gonads or roe of these fish during their reproductive season. The symptoms are characterized by headache, fever, dizziness, vomiting, colic, and diarrhea. Severe abdominal cramps, anuria, pallor, and prostration may also be present. Recovery is the rule, and no specific treatment is known.

Bacterial food poisoning from fish.—Some cases of fish poisoning may be of bacterial origin. Takashi Yasukawa (21) makes the following statement with reference to handling in Saipan:

> In this area the fish peddlers carry their wares on their heads in boxes (about 3 feet long by 2 feet wide by 6 inches deep) with 2 to 4 inch squares of wire screen in each side (for ventilation). The fish in the shops are so

covered with flies that it is hard to tell what species they are. Ice is never put on the fish as it is in Japan and consequently the fish are dried out, the color of the skin is faded, the elasticity of the muscles is lost, and the fish looks almost as if it had been exposed directly to the rays of the burning sun. Under such circumstances the protein of the flesh is decomposed and one feels deeply that eating such fish may give rise to so-called ptomaine poisoning [*sic*].

Obviously, there is need for more information on the biology of poisonous fishes as well as for careful pharmacological and chemical study of the poisons in toxic fish. The similarity of symptoms between mussel poisoning and some of the fish poisonings would suggest a common causative agent. The localization of the poison in fish needs study to evaluate the toxicity of the organs and flesh of poisonous fish. It has not been established whether the poison is ingested by fish in their food or whether it is manufactured in their metabolism.

AKEE POISONING

Akee poisoning is caused by eating the fruit of the akee tree (*Blighia sapida*). Jordan and Burrows (25, 26) have found that the seeds and pods of both ripe and unripe akees from Jamaica contain a substance which, upon ingestion, induces violent vomiting in young cats and *Macaca mulatta*. The arilli and placentae did not contain the substance. Their evidence suggested that the akee poison may be a glucoside. Lynch, Larson, and Doughty (27) have stated that the aril of the "yawning" akee is nontoxic. ("Yawning" is the term used to denote the splitting of the capsule, displaying the seeds and arils.) The arils are a white, fleshy substance in which the seeds are partly immersed and are seen when the mature pod splits longitudinally. The plant is firm, oily in texture, and has a nutlike flavor. In tropical America, southern Florida, and Jamaica it is valued as food. When tenderized by boiling in salt water and frying in butter, it is a rich protein supplement to the diet. Lynch, Larson, and Doughty noted that the arils of the "nonyawning" akee were toxic to rabbits. Wynn, Larson, and Doughty (28) stated that the arils of unripe fruit and the cotyledons of both ripe and unripe fruit have shown toxicity. The toxic principles are heat-stable and water-soluble and are not precipitated by the addition of ethyl alcohol. Wynn *et al.* found that the red and white cell counts of the blood are decreased in both dogs and rabbits with akee poisoning. There is a tendency for the blood chloride to increase. In rabbits there is a declining body temperature, followed by depression and death. At necropsy the kidneys are pale, the peritoneal cavity is moist, the lungs are congested, and the auricles of the heart are distended with venous blood. The stomach and small and large intestines are usually hyperemic. There may be subcutaneous hemorrhage in the tissues in the area of the external mammary blood vessels.

FAVISM

Favism, occurring mainly among Italians, is attributed to eating the fava bean or smelling the blossoms of the bean plant. A large Mediterranean population lives in the United States, and the fava beans are cultivated extensively in New York, New Jersey, Illinois, and California (29). The beans are a staple article of diet and are also imported as canned food from Italy. In 1,211 cases reported in the United States (30), 38 per cent developed after the inhalation of pollen and 62 per cent after the ingestion of raw or cooked beans. The yearly prevalence varies, and attacks occur most frequently after the ingestion of the first green beans of the season. Poisoning is more likely to occur in individuals who eat them often.

When fields of fava beans are in blossom, the inhalation type of the disease is prevalent. The pollen is said to be sticky and is not widely disseminated. The first symptom appearing after inhalation of substances originating from the flowers or plant of the fava bean is dizziness, sometimes reaching the stage of collapse. The attack may occur within a few minutes or some hours after exposure and is usually followed by the gradual appearance of headache, malaise, and nausea. Repeated yawning, vomiting, chills, pallor, and pain in the lumbar region are followed by high fever. The most specific symptoms are hemoglobinuria, which occurs within 5–40 hours, followed by icterus. T. McCrae and J. C. Ullery (31) reported a case with the following history:

December 12, 1932 J. C., a white man aged 53 was admitted to the Pennsylvania Hospital in a serious condition. He had a ghastly appearance due to a combination of jaundice and a curious ashen gray color, particularly of the face. He showed extreme weakness and complained of frequency of urination and the passage of black urine. Lesser complaints were of anorexia and constipation. He was intelligent and able to give a clear history. December 7, 1932, the man had eaten a very hearty meal, one of the principal constituents of which was cooked beans of which he had taken a large amount. An hour after the meal he began to feel marked weakness and was compelled to lie down. Two hours later he voided urine and noticed that it was very black. From this time until his admission to the hospital he was compelled to be in bed, the passage of black urine had continued and there had been a marked frequency of urination, usually about 19 times in the 24 hours. December 7 he had taken a large dose of Epsom salts and stated that blood was present in one of the stools after this. Shortly after the onset he began to have pain in the back, which had been constant. His weakness had increased markedly and since the second day of his illness he had not been able to get out of bed. On December 10th jaundice was noted for the first time and this apparently increased rapidly.

The patient volunteered the statement that he had similar attacks during his childhood in Sicily and associated his present illness with these. At the age of 7, while walking in the country, he passed a field of plants in full bloom. Soon after this he began to feel dizzy and weak, and he was able to walk a short distance only when he lost consciousness. He was found lying on the ground and was carried home, regaining consciousness later in the day. Following this he passed bloody urine for 3 or 4 days and felt marked weakness for about 10 days, after which he recovered his usual health. He stated that he had identical attacks each year from the age of 7 until he was 14, having one attack each year under the same circumstances. On each occasion he lost consciousness but did not know the exact duration of unconsciousness until the last attack, when he was told that it persisted for 15 hours. He came to the United States at the age of 14 and had had no similar trouble until his present illness. With the onset of this illness he at once recalled the experience of his childhood and associated the beans which he had eaten with the plants which had affected him when in flower. He thought the beans which he had eaten were the same as those which grew on the plants in Sicily.

McCrae and Ullery (31) mention that hypersensitiveness and anaphylactic shock can be produced by feeding the beans or injecting the protein of the bean first and later feeding the beans and also that the disease rarely occurs in persons who eat the beans regularly but often follows after the first eating of beans in a given year. The theory that this disease results from an allergy seems confirmed by a second case reported in the United States by Hutton (30). A man twenty-one years of age had eaten fava beans and became ill suddenly at a ball game. He complained of weakness, a yellowish tinge of the skin, and abdominal distress. The symptoms were similar to the previous case. The interesting feature here was the family history. The maternal grandmother had undergone several attacks of sudden weakness, accompanied by pallor, jaundice, and dark-brown, bloody urine. The acute picture lasted 3 or 4 days and was followed by rapid recovery. The mother and eldest brother had experienced similar attacks. The maternal great-grandfather, his sister, and all her children almost yearly suffered attacks in the spring during the fava season. A neighbor had given one of the maternal grandmother's children a few raw green fava beans with which to play. The child had eaten these beans and died within 24 hours from an attack after suffering collapse and jaundice.

Many cases of this disease in the United States are probably not recognized. Although there appears to be a hereditary basis for sensitization to this plant, the symptoms follow a definite pattern peculiar to this specific type of poisoning. Hutton states that a hereditary factor is present in 20 per cent of the cases. In certain families every member for generations had been reported severely affected. On the other hand, individual susceptibility varies, and specific people, after years of eating the beans without ill effect, may suffer a single severe attack. Ingestion of the beans by immune mothers may affect nursing infants. There is no sex predilection.

TREMATOL, MILK SICKNESS, OR SNAKEROOT POISONING

The disease called "milk sickness" is due to trematol ($C_{16}H_{22}O_3$) (32), which is one of the toxic constituents of white snakeroot, *Eupatorium urticaefolium,* found in the central states of the United States and of jimmy weed, *Aplopappus heterophyllus,* found in certain sections of western Texas, New Mexico, and Arizona. Cattle apparently will eat these weeds when grazing is scarce. White snakeroot is often abundant in heavily wooded areas. The poison produces "trembles" in cattle and milk sickness in man if he drinks milk or eats milk products from poisoned cows. Pasteurization does not destroy the poisonous properties. The symptoms of the disease in man are weakness or prostration, pernicious vomiting, severe constipation, and epigastric pain. The temperature is characteristically normal or subnormal. Muscular pains are common. There is great thirst, and the breath may have a distinct odor of acetone. The urine is scanty and may contain acetone. The cheeks are flushed, and there may be a marked redness of the lips and tongue. In fatal cases coma and convulsions precede death. In patients who recover, weakness persists for days, weeks, or even months, depending upon the initial severity of the illness.

The history of milk sickness is very interesting and is reported in an early paper by E. O. Jordan and N. M. Harris (33). This disease followed emigration in its westward march from North Carolina to Tennessee and Kentucky. It prevailed in various parts of Ohio, Indiana, and Illinois. The mother of Abraham Lincoln died of milk sickness at Pigeon Creek in southern Indiana in 1818. Whole villages in Illinois were depopulated by the ravages of this disease, which was responsible for nearly one-fourth of the deaths of pioneers and early settlers in Madison County, Ohio. In an old port in Dubois County, Indiana, in 1815, more than half the deaths were alleged to be due to milk sickness. The toll of livestock taken by "trembles" was also a great handicap to the pioneers. Trematol poisoning is known in the West as "alkali poisoning." Although the cause of the disease has been ascertained, sporadic cases still occur. G. H. Gowen (34) reported 21 cases in Illinois, in which there were 2 deaths. In every outbreak which he investigated, the animals which were responsible had been turned into a wooded area and were entirely dependent upon what they could forage.

MUSHROOM POISONING

Mushroom poisoning follows the eating of poisonous mushrooms which have been gathered in the woods and fields and mistaken for edible varieties. There are some seventy to eighty species of mushrooms that W. W. Ford (35) has found to be poisonous to man. The southern European population which has migrated to this country often confuses the poisonous ones with the European edible varieties. The differentiation of the various types of mushrooms is a matter for a trained mycologist and not for the layman.

The most poisonous mushroom is *Amanita phalloides*, sometimes called "white Amanita" or "deadly Amanita." In fact, two or three are sufficient to cause serious and fatal illness in the adult. Symptoms often appear within 15 minutes after eating the mushrooms but are sometimes delayed from 1 to 6 hours. This poisoning is characterized by salivation, excessive perspiration, a flow of tears, nausea, retching and vomiting, pain in the abdomen, and violent movement of the intestines, which causes profuse watery evacuations. The pupils are contracted. Respiration is often quickened and dyspneic. Dizziness and confusion of ideas are often noted. Coma may occur and death follow within 48 hours. In fatal cases, fatty infiltration with central necrosis is found in the liver, epithelial necrosis of the kidney, acute enteritis, and colitis. The uremic condition resulting from the kidney damage may be responsible for the symptoms. The case fatality in *A. phalloides* poisoning is from 60 to 100 per cent.

Dr. David Lewes (36) reported two cases of mushroom poisoning occurring in German prisoners of war in which the epidemiological features were carefully studied. He states:

> On the morning of September 11 they had gathered 'mushrooms' from a near-by wood; and the next day, after preparation, the fungi were boiled in water for three-quarters of an hour before being fried. The failure of the cooking 'mushrooms' to blacken a silver coin was considered proof that the meal would be safe; and each man ate approximately half a pound of mixed fungi. They found the meal most palatable and did not complain of ill effects until 9 and 12 hours later, respectively. In both cases initial symptoms consisted of severe vomiting, soon to be followed by intermittent attacks of griping upper abdominal pain and diarrhoea. Symptoms continued throughout the night, and on admission to hospital on September 13, 18 hours after ingestion, diarrhoea and vomiting had taken place fifteen times in H. W. and ten times in J. W.

A visit to the spot in the woods where the mushrooms were gathered with a trained botanist showed that, in unselected picking from the area concerned, *A. phalloides* constituted about 10 per cent of the fungi collected. *Amanita rubescens* (Warty Caps), a nonpoisonous variety, were plentiful, but no common mushrooms were found. It was estimated that in half a pound of uncooked fungi, each man ate one or at most two specimens of *A. phalloides*. This outbreak is of interest because it demonstrates that no reliance for safety can be placed upon the "silver-spoon test," and it also illustrates the danger in eating even a single specimen of *A. phalloides*.

Kobert in 1891 (37) isolated a powerful hemolytic substance from *A. phalloides* which he called "phallin." W. W. Ford (38) extracted the hemolytic substance and reported that it was of the nature of a toxin, since it acted upon the animal body after a definite latent period, produced lesions characteristic of bacterial intoxications in general, and induced immunity in susceptible animals by the inoculation of nonlethal doses. J. J. Abel and W. W. Ford (39) concluded that it was not a toxalbumin, as Kobert had supposed, but a nitrogenous glucoside, which is very sensitive to the action of heat and acids and less so to the action of alkalies. It is easily decomposed by acids to a pentose and a volatile base or bases, such as ammonia and methylamine. The latter found "phallin" in fresh specimens of *A. phalloides* and *A. citrina* and designated it "Amanita hemolysin." Since Seibert (40) failed to detect its presence in fresh extracts of *A. citrina*, the fungus may differ in its content of glucoside in various parts of the world. H. Schlesinger and W. W. Ford (41) studied the Amanita toxin and found that it could not be a protein, a glucoside, or an alkaloid. They make the following statement: "Nevertheless, since we are dealing with a conjugate sulfate which, on fusion with dry potassium hydrate, gives off pyrrol and indol we are led to conclude that Amanita-toxin, although not necessarily an indol derivative, is at least an aromatic phenol so combined with an amine group that it readily forms an indol or pyrrol ring."

Muscarine, which is a syrupy, alkaloidal-like substance, has been obtained in a crystallizable form as a hydrochloride from the mushroom *A. muscaria*. In its action it resembles pilocarpine, which stimulates the myoneural junctions. Treatment consists of stomach lavage, castor oil for eliminating any residual toxin from the gastrointestinal tract, and atropine sulphate (0.0005 gm.) subcutaneously.

The treatment of poisoning from *A. phalloides* has been reviewed by Binet, Leblanc, and Wellers (42). Rabbits poisoned with *A. phalloides* and treated with acetyl-*dl*-methionine to counteract liver damage lived longer than the controls which were untreated. These authors advise using both methionine and glucose, the latter to combat the hypoglycemia, in treating cases. Lewes (36) treated his patients with gastric and high colonic lavage with 1 per cent saline solution until the return fluid was clear. In 24 hours, 4–5 liters of 5 per cent glucose in normal saline were given intravenously and continued for 4 days, together with 15 units of soluble insulin and 10 mg. of vitamin K 4-hourly in an attempt to prevent or minimize liver damage. On the sixth day, unlimited glucose drinks and small quantities of citrated milk were substituted for the intravenous drip. Every 4 hours insulin injections combined with Vitamin K and vitamin B_1 12,000 units, and 10 ml. of 10 per cent solution of calcium gluconate parenterally were continued for a further 48 hours.

ERGOTISM

Ergotism is a rare type of poisoning, at least in the United States. It occurs as a result of eating a parasitic fungus, *Claviceps purpurea,* which causes a disease of rye and occasionally of other grains. The fungus grows in the grain as a blackish mass, which discolors the meal. A discussion of this poisoning is given by Barger (43). The essential features of ergot poisoning are listed in Table 2.

WATER-HEMLOCK POISONING

The water hemlock, *Cicuta maculata,* is often erroneously called "parsnip," "wild parsnip," or "wild carrot." Its habitat is in swamps, along irrigating ditches, and in wild meadows. Numerous references to the literature can be found in a paper by L. M. Gompertz (44), who describes an outbreak involving 17 boys. His description follows in part:

June 16, 1925, I was called to attend 17 boys, inmates of the New Haven County Home, who had been taken suddenly ill. The boys ranged in age from 9 to 13 years. All of the children in the institution had been dismissed from their classrooms at 3:30 P.M., apparently well, and immediately adjourned to their playground. At 5:15 the boys were in the dining room at their evening meal. The matron in charge observed that several of them refused their supper and appeared pale and sickly. Two of the children asked permission to leave the room, complaining of nausea, but before going very far fell to the floor in violent convulsions. About 20 minutes later, when I arrived, five children were in convulsions; twelve others were vomiting and appeared seriously ill. It was evident that the children were suffering from some form of poisoning, and I soon learned that they had partaken of a plant, the nature of which was unknown to me at the time. It later appeared, however, that in a plot of swamp land adjoining their playground water hemlock grew in abundance. While some of the boys had eaten the roots, the majority had partaken only of the leaves or flowers. It is noteworthy that the five boys who had eaten the root stock were very sick with accompanying convulsions, while the other twelve, who had eaten leaves or blossoms but no roots, did not have convulsions.

All 17 boys made complete recoveries.

In another outbreak in Coeburn, Virginia, 6 children, on April 15, 1951, were playing in a pasture and digging up the roots of what they thought were wild "white carrots" (*Daucus carota,* white carrot, or Queen Anne's lace). In reality, they were digging the roots of water hemlock (*C. maculata*) (45). Three children, aged four, ten, and eleven years, died, whereas those five, seven, and thirteen years of age survived. The eleven-year-old boy is known to have walked a mile to his home. The four-year-old was walking from the pasture toward home, and neighbors noticed she was crying as a result of falling. About 15 minutes later her mother found her in convulsions on the ground outside their home. It is thought that symptoms occurred less than 30 minutes after eating the root. All 6 children were taken to the Coeburn Hospital. Dr. J. D. Culbertson, physician in charge, stated that all 6 children were unconscious or disoriented when admitted. There was twitching of the eyes and facial muscles, no retraction of the head or neck, pupils dilated, possibly slight flushing of the skin, and later cyanosis. The heart rate was rapid until approaching death, and the heart tones were not good. All had convulsions and vomited. The treatment consisted of emptying the stomachs and giving large doses of atrophine. Deaths were thought to have occurred 3–4 hours after ingestion of the plant. The survivors were disoriented for a time, had some convulsions, and apparently could not focus well.

In Gompertz' (44) review of the literature he states that the poisonous component of *Cicuta* is a resin, which was first isolated and named "cicutoxin" by Boehm in 1876. Cutting the rootstock causes the exudation of an aromatic, yellowish, oil-like substance with an odor similar to parsnip. Cicutoxin is a clear, brown, sticky resin having an acid reaction. It is soluble in ether, alcohol, chloroform, and dilute alkalies.

POISON HONEY

A curious type of poisoning from honey has been described in the United States (8 cases in New Jersey in 1896), Brazil, Asia, and Africa. It appears to be common in the vicinity of the Black Sea. One of the earliest notices of poisoning from honey is that of Xenophon, the Athenian (434–354 B.C.), who in his account of the escape of the Greek army from the Persians (401 B.C.) tells of a food-poisoning outbreak among the Ten Thousand after they reached the Black Sea at Trapesus:

The soldiers camped in some mountain villages which they found well stocked with food and honey and observed a great number of beehives. All of the soldiers who ate of the honey became delirious and suffered vomiting and diarrhea. Those who had eaten a little behaved as though they were drunk, and those who had eaten much of the honey behaved like mad people. Some of these died. Large numbers lay on the ground, as though after a defeat and were despondent. Those alive the next day became lucid at about the same hour as they had eaten the honey the day before. On the third and fourth days they were able to get up. Most of them stated that they felt just as if they had been taking medicine [46].

The poison appears in the honey derived from certain nectar-bearing plants: varieties of azalea, rhododendron, oleander, and perhaps mountain laurel and palmetto (47). Honey from the flowers of the black locust has at times been toxic.

P. Pulewka (48) reviewed the literature concerning honey poisoning and reports that the distribution of poisonous honey is identical with that of poisonous rhododendron species. The toxin from the honey is referred to as "andromedotoxin," since it is found commonly in a genus of rhododendron called *Andromeda,* although apparently the poison is not limited to this genus. The chemical characteristics of andromedotoxin are: it is nitrogen-free, soluble in cold water to 2.81 per cent, in boiling water to 0.87 per cent, and the pH in water is approximately 7.0. Andromedotoxin is not precipitated by any alkaloid-precipitating agent, is soluble in alcohol and chloroform, dissolves with difficulty in ether and benzol, and is insoluble in petroleum ether. A red color develops when it is added to mineral acids. The toxin is not disintegrated by boiling in glacial acetic acid but is destroyed by prolonged boiling in a concentrated solution of tartaric or oxalic acid. Elementary analysis suggests the formula $C_{31}H_{51}O_{10}$.

The symptoms which follow in man after eating honey containing andromedotoxin are nausea, vomiting, diarrhea, dizziness, headache, temporary blindness, malaria-like fever attacks, fainting, and complete unconsciousness. Other symptoms reported are excitation, cramps, stomach and abdominal pain, burning sensations in the mouth and on the skin, and profuse sweating.

Pulewka studied the toxicity of honey samples from northern Anatolia by comparison with pure aconitin nitrate as a standard preparation. The test was based on the characteristic effect of andromedotoxin on the respiration of white mice. No toxin other than andromedotoxin was found in honey.

POTATO POISONING (SOLANINE)

The potato was not used as a food in Europe until the end of the sixteenth century, although it was introduced into Europe by Columbus. Medical literature before 1919 contains references to potato poisoning. Paul Khan (49) has reviewed this literature on solanine, a gluco-alkaloid of uncertain empirical formula, which is contained in all potatoes and other solanaceous plants. In large concentrations it is poisonous to animals; however, Khan has estimated that at least 8 kg. (17.6 pounds) would have to be consumed by man at one time to cause symptoms. Most of the cases of potato poisoning may be explained by bacterial agents or their products contaminating potatoes, and it may be concluded that no solanine poisoning hazard exists from the eating of potatoes.

RHUBARB POISONING

During World War I the use of rhubarb leaves as greens was recommended. In 1917 an editorial (50) appeared in this country, quoted here in part:

> Certain newspapers and magazines in this country are advocating the use of rhubarb leaves for greens. Advice to use the leaves as a substitute for spinach has been promulgated from at least one popular educational center. Because the rhubarb leaves contain certain substances—presumably oxalic acid—in sufficient quantity to make them toxic at times to some persons at least, and because disastrous results have followed their culinary use, the U.S. Department of Agriculture has issued a warning to housewives against using this portion of the plant for food.[3] How timely these instructions are is borne out by the report of a death from eating rhubarb leaves recently reported in the *Journal*.[4]

H. F. Robb (51) reports a case of rhubarb poisoning of a woman who had eaten rhubarb leaves fried and prepared as greens. Within 12 hours she had cramplike pains, which continued intermittently for a period of 36 hours or longer. Death occurred within 48 hours. A few hours before death the temperature was normal, the respiration 36 a minute, and the heartbeat 120 a minute. A brown bloody fluid was vomited, and a 6-month fetus was aborted. The blood from the placenta failed to clot. After death some blood coming from the nose also failed to clot.

3. U.S. Dept. Agriculture, Weekly News Letter, p. 2, May 23, 1917.
4. "London Letter," J.A.M.A., **68**:1928, 1917.

In the same year another report (52) was made of the poisoning of 9 people who had eaten canned rhubarb. These victims ranged in age from two to eighty-six years. Their symptoms, which came on uniformly within a 20-minute period, began about 2 hours after eating the rhubarb. Following the free use of a stomach pump, lime water, and castor oil, all recovered.

TUNG-NUT POISONING

Dr. J. Edward Balthrop (53, 54, 55) has reported 10 cases of tung-nut poisoning in children ranging from two to eleven years of age. The tung-nut tree, *Aleurites fordü, A. moluccana, A. trisperma,* and *A. montana,* has long been grown in China. *Aleurites fordü* has been introduced into the southeastern states. The tung tree grows rapidly, reaching a height of 40 feet. It is deciduous, shedding its leaves in the fall and remaining dormant during the winter months. The leaves are heart-shaped and large (*tung* is the Chinese word for "heart"). The tree flowers in the spring, and the flower is followed by a round green nut which appears at the end of shoots from the previous season. The pulpy exterior of the fruit covers a nutlike shell, inside of which are the seeds, usually about five. The ripe tung nut resembles a large walnut, and its seeds resemble a Brazil nut. Although the tung tree was not introduced into the United States until 1932, by 1948 the tonnage of nuts produced in the United States was 67,200. The oil of the tung nut is used in the paint industry. Balthrop (53) describes one outbreak as follows:

> On November 25, 1951, three colored males were brought in to the City Hospital emergency room with a history of having eaten tung nuts five hours previously. About 30 minutes after ingestion, they experienced violent nausea and vomiting, diarrhea and severe colicky abdominal pain. They were given lard by mouth, castor oil, and a mixture of milk and eggs at the onset of nausea, but they vomited it all back. Vomiting continued until one hour before being seen in the emergency room.

One child had eaten 5 tung seeds, one 6, and the third did not know how many he had eaten.

The symptoms common to all cases of tung-nut poisoning are nausea, vomiting, diarrhea, and abdominal cramps. Glycosuria was present in 9 out of 10 cases, and mydriasis in the same number of cases.

The nature of the toxic principle in tung nuts is unknown, although Balthrop considers a protein as the most likely toxic agent.

Tung nuts have decreased toxicity after treatment with hydrochloric acid, acetic acid, or magnesium sulphate.

The treatment recommended by Balthrop (54) is replacement of fluid and electrolytes, central nervous system stimulants, and magnesium sulphate by mouth. Pilocarpine was found to have no value in treatment either as a protective agent against poisoning or in treatment after poisoning had occurred.

REFERENCES

1. BULSTRODE, H. TIMBRELL. 39th Ann. Rep. Local Gov't Board, Supp. Rep. Med. Officer of Board, pp. 1–243. London: H.M. Stationery Office, 1909–10.
2. MEYER, K. F. Food poisoning, New England J. Med., **249**:765–73, 804–12, 843–52, 1953.
3. MEYER, K. F., SOMMER, HERMANN, and SCHOENHOLZ, P. J. Prevent. Med., **2**:365–94, 1928.
4. SOMMER, HERMANN, and MEYER, K. F. California State Dept. Pub. Health, Weekly Bull., **20**:53–55, April 26, 1941; with revision by Sommer through personal communication.
5. GIBBARD, J., COLLIER, F. C., and WHYTE, E. F. Canad. Pub. Health J., pp. 193–97, 1939.
6. MEDCOF, J. C., LEIM, A. H., NEEDLER, ALFREDA B., NEEDLER, A. W. H., GIBBARD, J., and NAUBERT, J. Bull. No. 75. Ottawa: Fisheries Research Board of Canada, 1947.
7. SOMMER, HERMANN, WHEDON, W. F., KOFOID, C. A., and STOHLER, R. Arch. Path., **24**:537–59, 1937.
8. WHEDON, W. F., and KOFOID, C. A. Univ. California Pub. in Zoöl., **41**: 25–34, 1936.
9. SOMMER, H., MONNIER, R. P., RIEGEL, B., STANGER, D. W., MOLD, J. D., WIKHOLM, D. M., and KIRALIS, E. S. J. Am. Chem. Soc., **70**:1015–18, March, 1948.
10. SOMMER, H., RIEGEL, B., STANGER, D. W., MOLD, J. D., WIKHOLM, D. M., and McCAUGHEY, M. B. J. Am. Chem. Soc., **70**:1019–21, March, 1948.
11. RIEGEL, BYRON, STANGER, D. WARREN, WIKHOLM, DONALD M., MOLD, JAMES D., and SOMMER, HERMANN. J. Biol. Chem., **177**:1–11, 1949.
12. STANGER, D. WARREN. Personal communication.
13. SOMMER, HERMANN. Personal communication.
14. AKIBA, TOMOICHIRO, and HATTORI, YASUZO. Jap. J. Exper. Med., **20**: 271–84, 1949.
15. AKIBA, TOMOICHIRO. Personal communication, June 12, 1952.
16. HALSTEAD, BRUCE W. Copeia, No. 1, pp. 31–33, 1953.
17. Letter to Capt. Harold F. Luke from Professor Ichiro Tokuyama, dated January 22, 1953.
18. HALSTEAD, BRUCE W., and BUNKER, NORMAN C. California Fish & Game, **39**:219–28, 1953.
19. GILMAN, ROBERT L. U.S. Nav. M. Bull., **40**:19–27, 1942.

20. Ross, S. G. M. J. Australia, **2**:617–21, 1947.
21. Poisonous fishes of the South Seas. Special Scientific Rep.: Fisheries, No. 25, p. 221. Washington: U.S. Dept. Interior, Fish and Wildlife Service, May, 1950.
22. Khlentzos, Constantine T. Am. J. Trop. Med., **30**:785–93, 1950.
23. Halstead, Bruce W. Personal communication.
24. Van Veen, A. G., and Latuasan, H. E. Docum. Neerl. et Indonesia de morbis tropicis, **2**:18–20, 1950.
25. Jordan, Edwin O., and Burrows, William. Proc. Soc. Exper. Biol. & Med., **31**:515–17, 1934.
26. ———. Am. J. Hyg., **25**:520–45, 1937.
27. Lynch, S. John, Larson, Edward, and Doughty, Donald D. Proc. Florida State Hort. Soc., **64**:281–84, 1951.
28. Wynn, Mark F., Larson, Edward, and Doughty, Donald D. Fed. Proc., Vol. **11**, March, 1952.
29. Luisada, A. Abstr., J.A.M.A., **117**:646, 1941.
30. Hutton, John E. J.A.M.A., **109**:1618–20, 1937.
31. McCrae, Thomas, and Ullery, J. C. J.A.M.A., **101**:1389–91, 1933.
32. Couch, J. F. J. Agr. Res., **40**:649, 1930.
33. Jordan, Edwin O., and Harris, Norman M. J. Infect. Dis., **6**:401–91, 1909.
34. Gowen, G. H. Illinois M. J., **74**:447–51, 1938.
35. Ford, W. W. J. Pharmacol. & Exper. Therap., **29**:305, 1926.
36. Lewes, David. Brit. M. J., **2**:383, 1948.
37. St. Petersburger med. Wchnschr., **16**:463, 471, 1891.
38. Ford, W. W. J. Infect. Dis., **3**:191–224, 1906.
39. Abel, J. J., and Ford, W. W. J. Biol. Chem., **2**:273–88, 1906–7.
40. Inaug. diss., Munich, 1893.
41. Schlesinger, H., and Ford, W. W. J. Biol. Chem., **3**:279–83, 1907.
42. Binet, Léon, Leblanc, Michele, and Wellers, George. Presse méd., Vol. **58**, No. 54, 1950.
43. New England J. Med., **306**:524, 1932.
44. Gompertz, Louis M. J.A.M.A., **87**:1277–78, 1926.
45. Personal communication from Dr. L. J. Roper, commissioner, Department of Health, Commonwealth of Virginia, April 27, 1951.
46. Jensen, L. B. Man's foods, p. 225. Champaign, Ill.: Garrard Press, 1953.
47. Pawlowsky, E. N. Gifttiere und ihre Giftigheit, pp. 476–78. Jena: Gustav Fischer, 1927.
48. Pulewka, P. Bull. Fac. Med., Istanbul, **12**:275–86, 1949.
49. Khan, Paul. A study of outbreaks of food poisoning alleged to be due to poisonous potatoes. Master's diss., University of Chicago, 1949.
50. J.A.M.A., **69**:122, 1917.
51. J.A.M.A., **73**:627, 1919.
52. Benson, H. W. J.A.M.A., **73**:1152, 1919.
53. Balthrop, J. Edward. Bull. of Staff, City Hospital, Mobile, Alabama, **21**:3–14, 1952.
54. Balthrop, J. Edward, and Gallagher, William B. Bull. of Staff, City Hospital, Mobile, Alabama, **21**:15–20, 1952.
55. Balthrop, Edward. South. M. J., **45**:864–65, 1952.

IV *Botulism*

Botulism is due to toxins formed by the growth of the botulinum microörganisms, usually in underprocessed home-canned foods. By the time that symptoms appear, the toxin has produced damage which often cannot be overcome by specific antitoxin therapy. War conditions in 1917–18 served as a stimulus to preserve more food. Then the danger of botulism was not recognized; hence considerable spoilage from underprocessing resulted, and an occasional outbreak of botulism occurred. Research to determine the cause of spoilage showed that the cold-pack method of processing foods for home canning, as recommended by the government, was entirely inadequate to prevent botulism. Coincident with outbreaks from home-canned products in 1918–19, commercially canned ripe olives and spinach were found to be responsible for cases of human botulism. The commercial canning industry, through the National Canners Association, established grants at several universities[1] for a study of the cause and prevention of botulism. Valuable contributions came from the United States Public Health Service. Aided by this research, commercial canners have practically controlled the disease in their field, as is attested by the fact that, with one possible exception (1), no outbreak of botulism has been reported since 1925 from commercially canned goods packed in the United States. Unfortunately, the record of home canning does not compare as favorably and constitutes the greatest problem in botulism today. The United States Department of Agriculture and state health departments have done commendable work in educating housewives to the danger of botulism and the need for safe processing of canned goods. The educational process is necessarily slow but nevertheless has probably been responsible for the decrease in outbreaks that has occurred. The number of annual outbreaks for the United States (2, 3, 4, 5) is

1. Harvard University, University of Chicago, Stanford University, and University of California.

tabulated in Table 3. When Canada is included, the figures are higher (6).

HISTORY

Botulism has been known in Europe for many years, with the first case recorded in 1735 (7). The term "botulismus" (*botulus*, a "sausage") was coined by physicians of southern Germany in the beginning of the nineteenth century to signify a type of food poisoning which was caused by the ingestion of spoiled sausages. Other names in use in the literature are "allantiasis," "ichthyosismus," and *Wurstvergiftung*. In the early years the term was restricted to sausage poisoning, but the symptom complex produced by sausage poisoning has been found to apply to poisoning involving other pre-

TABLE 3

Year	No. of Outbreaks	Year	No. of Outbreaks
1938.......	5	1946.......	7
1939.......	9	1947.......	12
1940.......	5	1948.......	7
1941.......	6	1949.......	4
1942.......	7	1950.......	3
1943.......	4	1951.......	9
1944.......	9	1952.......	2
1945.......	12	1953.......	7

served foods—smoked meat and fish and underprocessed canned vegetables and meat.

In 1895 Van Ermengem (8) succeeded in isolating a bacterium from ham which had caused the illness of 23 persons whose symptoms were those of true botulism. He proved that the poisoning in botulism is due to a toxin which is produced when the bacillus is grown upon a suitable culture medium.

A careful survey of the literature on botulism from early times up to 1918 has been made by Dickson (7), and the following ten years have been reviewed by Meyer (9). In December, 1919, following outbreaks of botulism resulting from the consumption of factory-preserved ripe olives, a commission was formed on the Pacific Coast. A subsequent investigation was sponsored by the National Canners Association, the Canners League of California, and the California

Olive Association. The purpose of the investigation was to determine the danger from botulism, its method of occurrence, and how it can be avoided and overcome. The report of the commission was included in a bulletin (10) entitled *The Epidemiology of Botulism,* published in 1922.

GEOGRAPHICAL DISTRIBUTION

Botulism has occurred throughout the civilized world. The reported outbreaks have been collected by Meyer (Table 4). Various foods have been implicated in outbreaks. For instance, in Germany most of the cases were from sausage. In Russia, on the other hand,

TABLE 4

Date	Geographical Location	No. of Reports	No. of Cases	Deaths
1735–1874.........	Württemberg	7	920	366
1789–1908.........	Europe	7	1,961	688
1886–1923.........	Germany	3	838	134
1897–1924.........	Prussia	2	397	65
1895–1906.........	Belgium	1	38	3
1901–1915.........	Denmark	2	4	1
1875–1924.........	France	4	21	3
1860–1926.........	Great Britain	4	75	10

outbreaks have occurred from salt herring, salt salmon, smoke-dried herring, dried sturgeon, and smoked sturgeon (11). One outbreak was caused by canned onions (shallots), which had been packed in Naples, Italy, and sold in the United States (12). Several cans in this shipment were found to contain potent toxin of *Clostridium botulinum.* Meyer (6) has collected data on 483 outbreaks (Table 5) occurring in the United States and Canada between 1899 and 1949.

TYPES OF FOOD INVOLVED IN OUTBREAKS OF BOTULISM

In Europe most botulism has followed the eating of preserved meats; in the United States home-canned vegetables have been responsible for the greatest number of cases. Geiger, Dickson, and Meyer (10) found that 62.3 per cent of the outbreaks in California were due to home-canned string beans, asparagus, corn, fruits (apricots and pears), and commercially packed ripe olives and spinach, while only 24.4 per cent were due to animal products, up to 1922. During 1940, data were collected on 15 outbreaks of botulism caused by home-canned goods, in which there were 30 cases and 14 deaths. This information came from newspaper reports, state health department reports, and the United States Food and Drug Administration. The foods which have been involved in outbreaks of botulism are listed in Table 6.

TABLE 5*

DATA COLLECTED BY K. F. MEYER CONCERNING BOTULISM
IN THE UNITED STATES AND CANADA (1899–1949)

Location	No. of Outbreaks	Location	No. of Outbreaks
California..........	184	Indiana..........	3
Washington........	61	South Dakota......	3
Colorado..........	31	Texas.............	3
Oregon............	26	Wisconsin.........	3
New York.........	25	Alabama..........	2
New Mexico.......	22	Arizona..........	2
Montana..........	13	Missouri..........	2
Nebraska.........	9	Nevada..........	2
Tennessee.........	9	Virginia..........	2
Wyoming..........	8	Arkansas..........	1
Idaho.............	7	Florida..........	1
Kentucky.........	6	Georgia..........	1
Illinois...........	6	Iowa.............	1
Canada...........	6	Maine............	1
Michigan..........	5	Maryland.........	1
New Jersey.......	5	Minnesota........	1
North Dakota.....	5	Mississippi.......	1
Ohio.............	5	Oklahoma........	1
Utah.............	5	Washington, D.C...	1
Massachusetts......	4	West Virginia......	1
Pennsylvania......	4		
Connecticut.......	3	Total.........	483

* 1,319 cases, with 851 deaths, or 64.5 per cent case fatality rate.

The degree of acidity and the nutrient value of the food are the important factors in determining the occurrence of growth of *Cl. botulinum*. The foul, rancid odor in some nonacid foods in which *Cl. botulinum* has grown has not been sufficiently emphasized. Owing to this odor, many foods are probably discarded and are not eaten. Canned meats, in particular, give off a foul odor as a result of the growth of *Cl. botulinum*. With the more acid foods with poorer nutrients for *Cl. botulinum*, the foul odor may not be so noticeable. This is the case in canned string beans. Wagenaar and Dack (13)

TABLE 6

FOODS WHICH WERE INVOLVED IN 462 OUTBREAKS OF BOTULISM
IN THE UNITED STATES BETWEEN 1899 AND 1947 (6)

Food	No. of Times	Preparation
Vegetables and fruits:		
String beans	97	Three commercially packed
Corn	47	One commercially packed
Beets	24	Two commercially packed
Spinach and chard	22	Ten commercially packed
Asparagus	21	Home-canned
Olives	14	Twelve commercially packed
Peas(?)	10	Home-canned
Figs	10	Home-canned
Beet greens	9	Home-canned
Chili peppers	9	Home-canned
Beans	7	Home-canned
Tomatoes	7	Home-canned
Mushrooms and mushroom sauce	6	Home-canned
Apricots	4	Home-canned
Okra	3	Home-canned
Pears	3	Home-canned
Pickles	3	Home-canned
Vegetables	3	Home-canned
Black-eyed Susan beans	2	Home-canned
Par-par	2	Home-canned
Soybean mash (Natto)	2	Home-canned
Pumpkin	2	Home-canned
Carrots	2	Home-canned
Green peppers	2	Home-canned
Green chili	2	Home-canned
Mixed salad beets(?)	1	
Okra and beans	1	Home-canned
Applesauce	1	Home-canned
Apricot butter	1	Home-canned
Beans and peppers	1	Home-canned
Cauliflower	1	Home-canned
Celery	1	Home-canned
Eggplant and green pepper	1	Home-canned
Mangoes	1	Home-canned
Persimmons	1	Home-canned
Pimiento	1	Home-canned
Okra, sourgrass, tomatoes	1	Home-canned
Squash	1	Home-canned
Succotash	1	Home-canned
Tomato catsup	1	Commercially packed
Tomato juice	1	Home-canned
Tomato relish	1	Home-canned
Turnips	1	Home-canned
Vegetable soup mixture	1	Home-canned
Eggplant	1	Home-canned
Lima beans	1	Home-canned
Pickled beets	1	Home-canned
Pickled string beans	1	Home-canned
Tomato or okra and corn(?)	1	Home-canned
Cucumber	1	Home-canned
Green tomato and green pepper	1	Home-canned
Peaches and pickles	1	Home-canned
Peaches	1	Home-canned
Chili	1	Home-canned
Shallots (Muscari)	1	Commercially packed in Italy

TABLE 6—*Continued*

Food	No. of Times	Preparation
Meat:		
Sausage..........................	6	Two commercially preserved
Ham (deviled ham included).........	5	One commercially preserved
Beef.............................	5	Home-preserved
Chicken..........................	3	Home-preserved
Blood sausage.....................	2	Home-preserved
Pork products....................	2	One commercially packed
Beef tamales.....................	1	Unknown
Buffalo meat.....................	1	Home-canned
Calf's head vinaigrette.............	1	Home-preserved
Frankfurter sausage................	1	Home-preserved
Pork and beans...................	1	Commercially canned
Liver sausage and blood sausage.......	1	Home-preserved
Tongue (pickled)...................	1	Home-preserved
Prepared food(?)...................	1	Home-canned
Bologna..........................	1	No details
Pickled pigsfeet...................	1	Home-prepared
Pimiento loaf.....................	1	Home-prepared
Lamb stew........................	1	Home-canned
Chili con carne...................	1	Home-prepared
Milk and milk products:		
Cheese and cottage cheese...........	5	Home-prepared
Milk (canned).....................	2	Commercially canned
Fish and seafoods:		
Salmon...........................	8	One commercially canned
Tuna.............................	7	Three commercially canned
Clams (clam juice and broth included)..	4	Commercially canned
Sardines (1 sardine and tomato sauce)..	4	Three commercially canned
Crab.............................	1	Home-canned
Fish (pickled).....................	1	Home-canned
Herring..........................	1	Home-canned
Sprats...........................	1	Commercially canned
Salmon eggs......................	1	Home-prepared
Miscellaneous:		
Antipasto (Italian).................	1	Commercially packed
Home brew.......................	1	Home-canned
Salad dressing (mustard)............	1	Home-canned
Unknown..........................	45	
Total...........................	462	

found that canned bread experimentally inoculated with the spores of three strains each of *Cl. botulinum* types A and B became toxic when the pH and moisture were suitable for growth. The toxic bread had the same appearance as nontoxic bread, but it had a rancid odor.

Slocum *et al.* reported an outbreak of botulism due to home-canned tomatoes (14). These tomatoes in a half-gallon jar were opened approximately 20 minutes before a meal. The housewife observed that they had a slightly "off-odor." The sample for bacteriological examination contained juice and seed and the solid tomatoes more or less disintegrated. The odor was that of butyric acid. In this material, type B toxin was demonstrated by feeding tests on guinea pigs and protection tests with type B antitoxin. Hall (15) reported 7 outbreaks of botulism in the Rocky Mountain region for the years 1929–32, one of which was caused by home-canned chili (a condiment sauce made with red peppers, tomatoes, and spices cooked in vinegar). The chili was spoiled, but no pH studies were reported. For the years 1932–36, Hall (16) reported 14 outbreaks of botulism in western United States. Chili was found to be responsible for 3. One type A and one type B *Cl. botulinum* were isolated in 2 instances. The pH of the incriminated food was not reported in any outbreaks.

The taste and smell given off by acid food products involved in 9 outbreaks of botulism have been summarized by Slocum, Welch, and Hunter (14). In 3 outbreaks in which home-canned pears were involved, the following changes were noted: in one case the pears were gassy and tasted "sharp"; in another the pears had a "peculiar taste"; in the third they were abnormal in odor and tasted very acrid. Three outbreaks involved home-canned apricots; in the first they were described as tasting "bitter," in the second as having a "peculiar taste," and in the third, "did not taste just right." In one outbreak home-canned tomato-onion chili was said to have had an "acrid taste" and to have smelled "strong."

Obviously, many people would not eat food which has a disagreeable odor or a bad taste; but, since there are degrees of tolerance among various individuals regarding the use of spoiled food, it is impossible to rely upon spoilage as a safeguard against botulism. Furthermore, evidence of spoilage has not been observed in all outbreaks. The majority of European strains of *Cl. botulinum* and the American type E strains causing human botulism are nonproteolytic and probably would give less evidence of spoilage. Often when foods are heated, the volatile products of spoilage are more easily detectable than when the food is eaten cold.

Food is frequently eaten by individuals who are aware that it is obviously spoiled. An illustration of this is recorded in an outbreak of botulism reported in South Dakota from home-canned string beans:

On September 14, 1936, in a small town in the northern part of the state, five people sat down to a meal consisting of potatoes, boiled bologna sausage, home-canned string beans, bread, butter, and coffee. The family consisting of C. A., owner of a small country hotel, his wife, M. A., and three boarders, A. J., J. R. R., and J. S., all sat down together at this meal. The beans, home-canned by the so-called cold-pack method, were noted to be slightly foamy and faintly rancid in odor upon opening the Mason jar in which they had been prepared. The landlady questioned their edibility but J. R. R. assured her they would be all right if rinsed off in cold water, whereupon she rinsed them at the kitchen sink through five changes of cold water and served them without further preparation. These beans had been purchased from a truck distributing vegetables from Minnesota and orginally offered for sale in the small store attached to the hotel. The remainder had been thriftily processed by the landlady. They were, therefore, wilted and stale at the time of canning. A boarder, J. S., was still able to detect a rancid odor when the beans were passed to him, so he took none of them. He described the odor as being somewhat like limburger cheese, but not strong enough to be offensive. He was the only one who ate none of the beans, although he ate heartily of all the other food; likewise he was the only one of the five to be alive and well 42 hours later [17].

EVALUATION OF BOTULISM HAZARD IN FOOD

Ingram and Robinson (18) have reviewed the literature on botulism in relation to acid foods and have concluded that unreserved acceptance cannot be given to the view that growth of *Cl. botulinum* can occur below pH 4.5, whether or not accompanied by microbes. They point out that there may have been an increase in acidity at the time of examining the food, whereas, at the time that growth and toxin production of *Cl. botulinum* occurred, the acidity may have been less.

Townsend, Yee, and Mercer (19) studied the inhibition of the growth of types A and B *Cl. botulinum* by acidification. They found that type A strains were either equally or more tolerant to acid than type B strains. There was an exception, however, in the case of fruit puddings with farina, where growth of a type B strain occurred at a much lower pH than with a type A strain without the production of toxin. They found that in several products toxin was present at the next pH level below the lowest at which gas was formed, which illustrates the fact that gas cannot be relied upon to tell whether growth and toxin production have occurred in a product. These authors found a pH of 4.6 a maximum for control purposes in products in which acidification is relied upon to inhibit the growth of *Cl. botulinum*. The lowest at which growth occurred in their experiments was pH 4.8 in pineapple rice pudding. In culture media they found that a higher pH was required for growth (corn-steep liquor pH 4.98; Wheaton's beef heart–casein medium pH 5.02; Yesair's pork medium pH 4.98).

Kadavy and Dack (20) experimentally inoculated the dough of canned bread with spores of *Cl. botulinum*, types A and B. The bread was baked and the cans sealed while hot. Some cans, in addition to the inoculum of spores of *Cl. botulinum*, received *B. mesentericus* and were stored at 22° and 38° C.; others were stored at 32° C. for 6 months with weekly cycling at 4.5° C. for periods of 16 hours. No toxin developed in bread with an initial pH of 4.9 and average moisture content of 34 per cent. Bread with an initial pH of 5.4 with 37 per cent moisture became ropy in a few instances and developed toxin after 6 months' storage. Further studies by Wagenaar and Dack (13) indicated that pH was the limiting factor determining the growth and toxin production of *Cl. botulinum*, types A and B. Canned bread with a pH of 4.8 and moisture not exceeding 34 per cent has been found safe from the hazard of botulism. Ingram and Robinson (21) studied changes in the viable count of cultures of *Cl. botulinum* in acid-buffered broths containing bread crumbs, after inoculation with approximately 10^4 vegetative cells or spores per milliliter. In 9 out of 10 experiments growth did not occur below pH 5.0; in the tenth it took place at pH 4.8.

Wagenaar and Dack (22) inoculated cheese spread with toxin-free spores of *Cl. botulinum* and packed the product in cans. Sixteen lots of cheese spread were prepared and stored at 32° C. for 6 months. Half of the spreads was prepared from cheese force-cured for 4 months, and the other half with cheese 1 month old. The spreads were processed to contain nearly 36 per cent moisture, with pH levels varying from 5.2 to 6.2 and salt concentrations of approximately 1.25 or 2.50 per cent. No botulinum toxin was demonstrated in any of 8 series of samples inoculated with 10,000 spores per gram of a mixture of 3 strains each of type A and type B spores. There was a gradual decrease in spores recoverable during the storage period.

Segalove and Dack (23) carried out experiments on dehydrated meat to determine the moisture content and length of incubation necessary for *Cl. botulinum* type A to grow. Growth and production of toxin occurred in 48 hours on samples containing 60 per cent moisture. It occurred after 1 week of incubation at 37° C. in samples containing 40 per cent moisture. Samples containing 30 per cent moisture or less showed no evidence of toxin even after incubation at 37° C. for as long as 9 months. In a study of dried whale meat with a moisture content well below 30 per cent, Robinson, Pugh, and Selbie (24) found low anaerobic spore counts and low aerobic bacteria counts in 44 samples.

Steinke and Foster (25) inoculated liver sausage with spores of *Cl. botulinum* type A, stuffed it into Saran wrap, and incubated it at 30° C. Toxin was formed in 9–23 days, when the sausage contained 2.5 per cent salt, 0.1 per cent sodium nitrate, and 5,000 spores per gram and, when held at 18° C. and 10° C., did not become toxic in 90 and 205 days, respectively.

Wagenaar and Dack (26) studied the effect of salt, pH, disodium phosphate, and sodium citrate added to surface-ripened cheese which had been experimentally inoculated with the spores of type A or B. The sodium chloride concentration in cheese spread affects growth and toxin production of *Cl. botulinum*. Two and one-half per cent disodium phosphate reduced the amount of sodium chloride required for inhibition equivalent to the effect produced by increasing the sodium chloride level in the cheese approximately 1.0 per cent. Sodium citrate in a 2.5 per cent concentration was less inhibitory than the same amount of disodium phosphate. Growth and toxin production of *Cl. botulinum* occurred in brine concentrations up to approximately 8 per cent. Raising the pH level of this cheese from 5.7–6.2 to nearer neutrality (pH 6.6–7.2) by the addition of concentrated sodium hydroxide did not improve growth and toxin production of the *Cl. botulinum* organisms. In one mold-ripened cheese, raising the pH to this level enhanced the growth and toxin production of *Cl. botulinum*.

SYMPTOMS OF BOTULISM

A number of symptoms may result from the ingestion of food containing botulinum toxin. In some individuals the symptoms involving the central nervous system, which are characteristic of botulism, are preceded by an acute digestive disturbance and vomiting. These upsets are not due to peculiarities in the food items, since many individuals eating the same food will exhibit different reactions. In the outbreak described by Hunter and others (17), 3 of 4 individuals who had eaten less than a teaspoonful of the beans had no digestive upset. In an outbreak in Grafton, North Dakota (27), in which 16 individuals ate home-canned (cold-pack method) mixed diced carrots, peas, and cut string beans, 13 died. The 3 who survived had been drinking homemade beer and wine and had vomited before, during, or just after lunch. Some of the victims vomited later, but not until after absorption of a fatal dose of botulinum toxin. The author had the opportunity to observe botulism (12) in 2 men who ate sandwiches made with canned Italian onions, which had been packed in Naples, Italy. The onions were later shown to contain type B botulinum toxin. One man died, and the other, who survived, stated that he was nauseated after eating and took a large dose of Epsom salts. He had absorbed enough botulinum toxin, however, to cause diplopia and difficulty in swallowing. The latter symptom was well illustrated by the patient's statement that he had to drink a pint of coffee to enable him to swallow a doughnut, which was his customary breakfast.

Nausea and vomiting usually come on within 24 hours and appear to bear a relationship to the degree of spoilage and to the amount of incriminated food eaten. Diarrhea may occur early, but in the later stages of the disease constipation is present. This is illustrated in the outbreaks described by Dickson (7). In outbreak No. 1, 5 persons who had eaten spoiled apricots did not develop nausea or vomiting, owing probably to the feeble growth of *Cl. botulinum* and to the small amount of toxin. In outbreak No. 2, no nausea, diarrhea, or vomiting occurred when only two spoonfuls of spoiled home-canned corn were consumed. In outbreak No. 4, a woman opened a jar of home-canned string beans and, noting an unpleasant odor, tasted one of the pods. She developed nausea after 2 days, at which time neurological symptoms had developed. In outbreak No. 6, a woman noticed that one of a number of jars of string beans, which she had canned 2 weeks before, was leaking. She tasted one of the pods and noted that it was "slightly sharp." Subsequently, she threw out the contents of the jar. She developed no nausea or vomiting. In all except the first-mentioned outbreak, very small amounts of the food in question were eaten. In contrast to these, in outbreak No. 3 a woman opened a jar of home-canned asparagus and drank the juice. She became nauseated and vomited in about 6 hours. In an outbreak previously referred to, which was reported by Hunter and others (17), the person who ate less than a spoonful of the incriminated string beans had no symptoms of nausea or vomiting, while 3 other adults who had eaten an average helping of the beans became nauseated and vomited.

The typical symptoms of botulism usually appear within 12–36 hours, although as short a period as 2–4 hours is mentioned (10) and a much longer period may elapse. In the outbreak of botulism in Grafton, North Dakota, in which 13 of the 16 persons died, the last person affected developed symptoms 108 hours after the meal. During the first 3 days of his illness he went about town, attended the funerals of his fellow-victims, testified before the coroner's hearing, and was interviewed by several doctors, who thought that his symptoms might be psychic in origin (28). He refused hospitalization, but on the fourth day after the onset of symptoms, while running down an alley in response to a volunteer fire call, he fell down and was unable to rise. He was picked up by friends and taken to the hospital. At this time he exhibited marked muscular weakness and was unable to turn in bed without great difficulty. The sensorium was clear until death, which came from respiratory paralysis. In other words, this patient was active for about 8 days before hospitalization, his symptoms developed slowly, and he did not die until 10 days after ingesting the botulinum toxin.

When gastrointestinal symptoms are present, the patient may complain of burning and distress in the abdomen. Although constipation may be preceded by diarrhea, it often occurs early and is usually present throughout the illness. There is no colicky pain or tenderness in the abdomen. In the majority of cases the earliest symptom is a peculiar lassitude or fatigue, which is sometimes associated with dizziness or headache and often attributed to constipation.

Such disturbances as double vision (diplopia) occur early as a result of paralysis of some of the extraocular muscles. The third cranial nerve is involved. Blepharoptosis, mydriasis, and loss of reflex to light stimulation are present with the diplopia. Impaired function of the external rectus muscle appears. Photophobia, nystagmus, and vertigo are occasionally recorded. Difficulty in swallowing occurs early, and difficulty in speech is observed later. Sometimes the throat is described as feeling constricted. The tongue is coated and swollen and moves with difficulty. Paralysis of the pharyngeal muscles occurs in fatal cases, with regurgitation of fluids through the nose and mouth. There is usually considerable dryness of the mouth.

The muscles of the neck are often weakened. Dickson, in outbreak No. 7, thus quotes a man who was convalescing from botulism: "When putting on my shoes I found it very difficult to get my head and neck back to normal position, and in many cases it was necessary for me to push my head up with my hands." Some patients complain of muscle inco-ordination, which may be due to visual disturbances. Others have difficulty moving around, and some even experience falls.

There is no retention of urine, although the amount may diminish, since many patients cannot swallow and proper fluid balance is not maintained. The temperature is normal or subnormal. When it is elevated, a bronchopneumonia or aspiration pneumonia may have developed. The pulse may be normal but often becomes rapid in the later stages, and a Cheyne-Stokes respiration has been observed before death. The blood pressure is usually normal, and no abnormalities have been found in the blood cells as regards type or number.

Death is usually due to respiratory failure. The heartbeat has often been detected for some minutes after respiration has ceased.

One feature of botulism is that the patients' mentalities are lucid until a short time before death. Although they may not be able to speak, those affected can often express themselves in writing.

The duration of illness in fatal cases is usually from 3 to 6 days after ingesting the poisonous food. For example, in a series of 173 fatal cases, 18 patients died within 48 hours, 117 (67.6 per cent) died within 3–6 days, and 1 survived for 26 days (10).

The symptoms produced by all the toxins are similar, despite biochemical differences between strains.

TREATMENT

The treatment of botulism is unsatisfactory at best. Obviously, the sooner botulism is recognized, the better the opportunity for the physician to help those individuals who have eaten less of the poisonous food and have not manifested symptoms early. Unfortunately, when the disease is recognized, there is usually no antitoxin available locally. Therefore, more time elapses, during which absorption of toxin and irreparable damage to tissues take place.

The fact that symptoms may appear within 24 hours when potent toxin is administered and that antitoxin therapy is of less value, once symptoms have appeared, is illustrated by experiments carried out upon monkeys by the author (29). As shown in Table 7, monkey No. 1 not only showed symptoms early but died in 18 hours as the result of a potent dose of toxin. Other monkeys Nos. 2, 3, 6, and 9 died or survived, depending upon the amount of toxin given. Monkeys Nos. 4, 5, and 10 were given antitoxin intravenously after symptoms has occurred, but died.

On the other hand, in one outbreak which occurred in Ohio, the administration of antitoxin appeared to be of definite value in therapy (30). In Russia, Velikanov and Kolesnikova (31) treated 227 cases of botulism. Of these, 146 were treated with a specific serum, and 76 were not given serum. The treatment of the remaining 5 cases was not indicated. The mortality in the first group was 18 per cent and in the second group 93 per cent. Analysis of the first group revealed that serum was administered in the agonal stage to several of the 26 who died. Thus, as previously concluded, the effectiveness of the specific serum depended upon its early administration, as well as the dosage. The authors advise a dosage of from 50 to 60 ml., which is to be repeated within 5–10 hours if no improvement is noted. They found that the serum is best given intramuscularly. In 2 apparently hopeless cases the intraspinal introduction of 20 ml. of the serum had a remarkable effect. It was their conclusion that specific serum therapy in botulism gives the best curative results.

Since botulinum antitoxin is the only known specific therapeutic agent for botulism, its use should be encouraged, even though the disease is advanced. Moreover, although botulinum toxin is not formed in toxic food after ingestion, damage to the body may con-

TABLE 7

Effect of Botulinum Type A Toxin and Homologous Antitoxin on Monkeys

Monkey No.	Wt. (Kg.)	Ml. of Toxin Fed	No. of M.L.D. (Mouse)	Hours Elapsing before Symptoms Appeared	Toxin in Blood	Ml. of Antitoxin*	Time of Death after Feeding (Hours)	Comments
1....	.....	2	400,000	17.5	+	0	18	No toxin found in stomach but was demonstrated in large intestine in 1–2,000 dilution
2....	.....	0.1	20,000	22.75	+	0	24	Ate hearty meal 20.5 hours after feeding; no toxin found in the stomach
3....	3.5	1	2,000+	45	0	0	51	No toxin demonstrated in stomach, small intestine, or large intestine
4....	3.0	1	2,000	102	......	{3(IV), 1(SC)}	124	Given 20 ml. of 10 per cent glucose intraperitoneally after 121 hours
5....	2.6	2	20,000	53.5	0	2(IV)†	62	Fed 100 ml. cream with toxin; given 0.25 gm. barbital by mouth after 55.5 hours; given 0.25 gm. barbital intravenously after 57 hours
6....	3.5	2	20,000(?)	71	0	0	73.25	Given 0.18 gm. barbital intravenously after 73 hours
7....	.....	0.1	200+	0	......	0	Lived	Blood was tested for antitoxin 32 days later; the mouse receiving 1 ml. serum plus one M.L.D. of toxin died after a longer time than did the control mouse, which received the toxin alone
7....	.....	5	3,500	Not observed	+	0	38.5	Fed 50 days after previous feeding
8....	2.6	0.01	20+	0	......	0	Lived	No symptoms
8....	.....	1	10,000	....	......	....	Lived	Fed 14 days after first feeding; showed symptoms which consisted of general weakness; blood was tested for antitoxin 18 days later; the mouse receiving 1 ml. of serum plus one M.L.D. of toxin lived a day longer than did control mouse
8....	2.9	0.1	200+	0	......	0	Lived	Fed 75 days after last feeding; toxin 10 days old
8....	2.9	2	40,000	19	+	0	27.5	Fed 4 days after last feeding; first symptoms consisted of general weakness; considerable effort was required for the animal to move
9....	3.5	0.1	200+	0	......	0	Lived	No symptoms
9....	.....	2	40,000	Not observed	+	0	18	Fed 4 days after last feeding
10....	3.9	2	40,000	19.5	+	3(IV)	25	Fed 7.5 gm. MgSO₄ in water 8 hours after feeding toxin; part of the MgSO₄ was vomited, and 5 more gm. were fed; 20.5 hours after feeding toxin, the monkey was fed 100 ml. of strong coffee; after taking 5 ml. of blood for toxin titration, antitoxin was given

* The antitoxin was given when symptoms appeared. (IV) = intravenous; (SC) = subcutaneous.

† This antitoxin was given 2.5 hours after symptoms appeared.

tinue as the result of a gradual absorption of toxin as long as the latter remains in the intestinal tract. It is recommended that large doses of polyvalent antitoxin be given when the specific type of organism is unknown. In the therapy of botulism, at least 50,000 units should be given intramuscularly after the patient has been tested for hypersensitiveness and, if necessary, desensitized. Watson (32) recommends giving antitoxin intravenously in large doses in 1,000–1,500 ml. of 5 per cent glucose in normal salt solution with 8 minims of epinephrine added. When small amounts of toxin are ingested because of laboratory accidents in pipetting, 5,000 units of the antitoxin may be given. In the author's experience, 2 accidental cases have been so treated with no untoward effects. In addition, enemas are recommended for washing out the colon to eliminate any toxin which might be retained because of constipation.

In addition to specific treatment with antitoxin, it is important that other measures be taken. When symptoms of botulism develop, symptomatic treatment is directed chiefly to the maintenance of the fluid balance of the body. Pharyngeal paralysis, frequently an early symptom, necessitates the administration of fluids parenterally. Even though the patient may be willing to attempt to take fluids or food by mouth, this ought to be discouraged because of the danger of aspiration pneumonia. Measures should also be taken to avoid the aspiration of saliva. The patient should be kept in quiet, restful surroundings and encouraged to avoid even the slightest unnecessary muscular exertion.

In some cases artificial respiration has sustained life, but only for as long as it was continued. The Drinker respirator has been used in several cases (1, 33, 34) but not with great success. Orton (35) reported 3 cases of botulism in which 2 died and a tracheostomy was performed on the third. After tracheostomy, mucus was suddenly expelled from the trachea, and gradual improvement followed. Saline glucose solution (1,000 ml. containing 200,000 units of penicillin and 30,000 units of botulinum antitoxin) was given intravenously to the patient soon after admission to the hospital.

In outbreaks of botulism in which several individuals have eaten food containing toxin, those who may have only tasted the food or eaten sparingly of it usually do not develop symptoms until considerably later than those who have eaten generously of it. There is considerable experimental evidence in favor of antitoxin for prophylactic treatment in such cases.

In addition to the effect of dosage in determining the time of onset of symptoms, there may be another factor to consider in explaining delayed symptoms. Gastrointestinal upsets which occur early in some patients may cause the toxin to remain only a short time in the stomach and small intestine. Once the toxin is in the colon, it may remain for some time, since constipation is the rule in many instances. In the circumstance of a long stay in the colon, there may be slow and gradual absorption until a sufficient quantity is absorbed to produce symptoms. This contention is borne out by experimental work with type A botulinum toxin in the monkey (36) and is further supported by the fact that botulinum toxin is not readily destroyed in intestinal contents. Thus toxin has been found to persist in isolated loops of ileum in the dog (37) for at least 12 days.

Like man, the guinea pig is highly susceptible to botulinum toxin. The following experiment (38) suggests that the greatest absorption of the toxin probably occurs in the upper part of the intestinal tract. Two guinea pigs were given an intracecal injection of 1 ml. of type A botulinum toxin, of which 0.001 ml. constituted a minimum lethal dose for mice injected intraperitoneally. One animal died on the seventeenth day, with typical symptoms of botulism, whereas the other guinea pig survived. Seventeen days later the animal which survived was fed the same amount of toxin (1 ml.) of the same lot, which, in the interim, had been stored in the refrigerator. This animal developed symptoms of botulism on the fourth day and died on the seventh day.

MORTALITY AND PATHOLOGY

The mortality from botulism is approximately 65 per cent in the United States, but it is low in Europe. In many outbreaks all who eat the incriminated food die. Death hinges upon the amount of botulinum toxin ingested and absorbed. When a large dose is taken, the onset of symptoms occurs in a short time. According to Geiger and others (10), symptoms appeared within 48 hours after ingestion of the poison in 85 per cent of 173 fatal cases. Although vomiting shortly after eating may eliminate the toxin, this does not usually happen for several hours. During the lapse of this time a fatal dose of botulinum toxin is often absorbed.

There are no gross lesions which characterize botulism after death. When death occurs in less than 48 hours, microscopic changes are often not observed. In patients in whom the progress of the intoxication has not been too rapid, cellular thrombi have been found (10) in the meningeal veins. The thrombi consist of dense masses of fibrin arranged in thick bands, with many polymorphonuclear leukocytes enmeshed between the strands (7). Although the thrombi when present may suggest that death was caused by botulism, they cannot be considered pathognomonic of botulism (10).

MODE OF ACTION OF BOTULINUM TOXINS

Dickson and Shevky (39, 40), Edmunds and Long (41), and Bishop and Bronfenbrenner (42) have noted that botulinum toxin acts somewhat like the drug curare upon the end-plates of the nerves and appears to affect the myoneural junction of the skeletal motor apparatus. Guyton and MacDonald (43) have pointed out a fundamental difference between curare and botulinum toxin, namely, that acetylcholine or nicotine injected intra-arterially causes contraction of muscle poisoned by botulinum toxin but not in muscle poisoned by curare. Small amounts of either type A or type B toxin decrease the synthesis of acetylcholine in both in vivo and in vitro experiments.

The effect of botulinum toxin on the electromyogram of the guinea pig and cat was studied by Masland and Gammon (44). Local botulism was produced when the toxin was injected intramuscularly and was evidenced by muscle flaccidity without fibrillation. Prostigmine did not reverse the action of the toxin, as is the case in curare poisoning. Torda and Wolff (45) found that choline acetylase is strongly inhibited by the toxin and thought this might explain how the toxin produces neuromuscular block. In contrast, Burgen et al. (46) found that botulinum toxin exerted no inhibitory effect on the acetylation of choline by either fresh or acetone-dried rat brain. In their studies of botulinum toxin in a phrenic nerve–diaphragm preparation from the rat they were unable to localize with certainty the site of action of the toxin. These workers suggested that there is an interaction of toxin with the fine unmyelinated motor nerve fibers entering the end-plate region, thus causing a block in the transmission of the nerve impulse. This seems unlikely, since Ambache (47–49) has shown that botulinum toxin acts preferentially upon the cholinergic fibers that are myelinated up to their endings. Ambache (47) injected botulinum toxin into isolated intestinal segments of mice and rabbits and found a loss of peristaltic activity and of motor response to nicotine. There is a gradual loss of the stimulating action to small doses of nicotine; inhibition is produced instead of stimulation. This change in the nicotine response of the intestine after local injection of the botulinum toxin is explained by the selective affinity of the toxin for the cholinergic nerve endings, leading to the abolition of the stimulating action of small doses of nicotine and unmasking the response of the ganglion cells giving rise to adrenergic fibers which are not affected by the toxin. Ambache (48) in a subsequent study examined the susceptibility to botulinum toxin of a number of different nerves of the autonomic system of the cat. He produced paralysis of the ciliary ganglion by retrobulbar injections of toxin and located the lesion in the preganglionic fibers. Later he (49) studied the effect of toxin injected into the superior cervical ganglion on one side in 16 cats. The integrity of the ganglionic transmission was examined 20–48 hours later in the following two pathways: (*a*) that to the dilator papillae and (*b*) that to the nictitating membrane; and it was found that, with adequate doses of toxin, a complete preganglionic paralysis occurred in the papillo-dilator pathway, but some nictitating membrane synapses were able to withstand the paralytic action of the toxin, even in large amounts. Stover, Fingerman, and Forester (50) determined the electric reactions of sartorius muscle–sartorius nerve of the frog poisoned with type A botulinum toxin. They concluded that the paralytic action of botulinum toxin is due primarily to a depression of the motor end-plate mechanism and not to a blocking of the terminal nerve fibers. They suggested that the mechanism whereby acetycholine is released is probably inhibited.

Brooks (51) studied the question of whether botulinum toxin acted by blocking the motor nerve terminals just proximal to the site of acetylcholine release or whether the toxin interferes with the process of release itself. He used the cat's gracilis muscle *in situ* and the guinea pig's excised serratus muscle mounted in a bath of oxygenated Ringer-Locke solution. Brooks concluded that type A botulinum toxin produced neuromuscular paralysis by interfering with conduction in the terminal twigs of motor nerves, close to or at the points of final branching but proximal to the site of acetylcholine release.

Davies *et al.* (52) described the similarity between the action of the toxins of *Cl. tetani* and of *Cl. botulinum* on the neuromuscular mechanism of the rabbit's iris. Both toxins injected into the anterior chamber of the eye cause a prolonged paralysis of the sphincter pupillae muscle, which becomes unresponsive either to light reflex or to direct stimulation of the third cranial nerve. The paralyzed irises contract under the stimulus of small doses of acetylcholine or carbachol, showing that the toxin action is not on the nerve fibers themselves. Neither toxin affects the adrenergic mechanism of the dilator pupillae, which remains normally responsive to electrical stimulation of the sympathetic supply. These workers pointed out that, in addition to the paralytic action on the cholinergic mechanism of the iris, tetanus toxin leads to exaggerated activity of central nervous structures when injected into the spinal cord or medulla. However, when they injected type A botulinum toxin into the medulla oblongata and sciatic nerve trunks of rabbits, no local neurological disturbance occurred.

VARIATIONS IN SUSCEPTIBILITY OF DIFFERENT ANIMAL SPECIES TO BOTULINUM TOXIN

Although the toxins produced by the various types of *Cl. botulinum* cause similar symptoms, it has been found that different animal species vary in their susceptibilities to the toxins of the various types. Burgen, Dickens, and Zatman (46) determined the LD_{50} of type A and type B toxins by intraperitoneal injection into 200-gm. white rats. They found the LD_{50} for the rat of type A toxin to be equal to 25 mouse LD_{50}, and for type B toxin the LD_{50} for the rat to be equal to 10,000 mouse LD_{50}. Moll and Brandly (53) fed concentrated botulinum toxin of type A and type B to mink and noted that 20–80 million mouse M.L.D. (intraperitoneally) were required to produce symptoms of botulism. Quortrup and Holt (54) demonstrated that mink were highly susceptible to type C botulinum toxin. Dinter and Kull (55) described 3 outbreaks of botulism in mink on farms in Sweden, which were caused by *Cl. botulinum* type C. Kull and Moberg (56) established that the cause of death in 12 of 22 minks which came from different mink farms in Sweden was type C botulism. Wagenaar, Dack, and Mayer (57) found that mink remained healthy when fed meat cultures of *Cl. botulinum* types A, B, and E but developed symptoms and died when fed type C meat cultures. On the other hand, monkeys (*Macaca mulatta*) were susceptible when fed meat cultures of *Cl. botulinum* types C and E. Samples of mink food prepared at a mink ranch were inoculated with toxin-free spores of *Cl. botulinum* types A, B, C, and E. In these food samples, incubated at 30° C. for 24 hours, no botulinum toxin developed. Control beef heart medium when similarly inoculated became toxic in 24 hours with types A and C but not with types B and E. Toxin of type C developed when spores of this type of *Cl. botulinum* plus fly larvae or eggs of *Lucilia illustris* were added to the mink food and incubated at 30° C. for 24 hours. Thus the importance of sanitation in preventing the multiplication of fly larvae in mink food is clearly evident.

Cartwright and Lauffer (58) established a method for the assay of type A botulinum toxin in goldfish. They found that when 10 fish were inoculated per dilution with a tenfold dilution interval, the end-point distribution had a standard deviation of about 0.24 log units. The end-points were strongly temperature-dependent, decreasing about a hundred fold for a temperature decrease of 15° C. The end-point in fish at 34° C. is approximately the same as for mice.

LABORATORY DIAGNOSIS OF BOTULISM

The laboratory diagnosis of botulism is not always easy, as the suspected food may have been discarded and only necropsy material may be obtainable. Sometimes the food is fed to chickens, which have subsequently developed limber-neck (fowl botulism) and died. In fact, in studying outbreaks of botulism, it is advisable to inquire: (1) What items of food were fed to chickens? (2) If any were fed, were the chickens made ill? (3) Were there any deaths? It has been reported (59) that chickens, although susceptible to type A toxin when ingested, are highly refractory to type B toxin administered by the same route. However, in a subsequent report by other investigators (10) chickens were reported killed from eating food containing type B toxin. A sample of the food suspected of causing botulism may be simply a small portion remaining in a container or a few dried fragments rescued from the garbage; it may be vomitus, stomach washings, or portions of the bowel taken at necropsy; it may be another can from the same stock of canned food. In the case of the onions (12) which were canned in Naples, Italy, many of the unopened cans from the same lot contained viable *Cl. botulinum* type B as well as potent toxin. On the other hand, in the Loch Maree tragedy in the western Highlands of Scotland, in which 8 people died who ate potted wild-duck paste (60), over a million jars had been packed that year, and apparently only one contained *Cl. botulinum* organisms and toxin. Dauer (2) reported a single case of botulism caused by a commercial cheese spread in 1951. The author investigated this outbreak and found that this instance was similar to the Loch Maree outbreak, in that only one jar out of several million contained type B toxin.

Strains of *Cl. botulinum* types A and B may often produce gas and give rise to "swells" in food packed in tin cans, but not invariably. A systematic bacteriologic and toxicologic study was made (61) on 346 cans of commercially packed food products of both plant and animal origin. These foods were artificially inoculated with washed and heated spores of *Cl. botulinum* and incubated at room temperature and at 35° C., or both, for periods extending from 10 days to 12 months. Corn, peas, salmon, sweet potatoes, and pumpkin were found to undergo spoilage quickly and to develop very toxic decomposition products. Asparagus and beets became spoiled and toxic without swelling, and the spoilage was not sufficient to warn the consumer. Growth and toxin production of *Cl. botulinum* were found to be irregular in spinach; when growth occurred, it might or might not give rise to "swells." In some spinach a spoiled, butyric acid or cheesy odor was evident. Bulging occurred in 50 per cent of the inoculated cans of string beans. Toxins have frequently been found in cans which have normal odor and contain firm pods of natural color.

In laboratory diagnosis one cannot rely on odor or gross signs of spoilage in previously unopened containers as evidence of the presence of toxin. It is a wise plan to determine the pH of the product in question, because much can often be learned from such data about factors limiting the growth of the organism. Growth is uncertain at pH 5.4 or lower, although it depends somewhat on the nutritive value of the food to *Cl. botulinum*. The glass-electrode potentiometer is useful in making determinations in samples of food that are highly turbid or colored.

Obviously, the presence or absence of toxin in a specimen submitted for examination is of great importance. The presence of toxin is determined as follows: The sample is ground in a mortar with sterile sand and saline as needed. The suspension is centrifugalized at high speed for 1 or 2 hours. One-half-milliliter portions of the supernatant fluid are then withdrawn and injected intraperitoneally into mice, some of the mice being protected with types A and B antitoxins. If all animals should die with symptoms simulating botulism, type E antitoxin should be used in a second series of tests, since outbreaks of this type have been described in man. Filtration through a Berkefeld filter is purposely avoided, inasmuch as it reduces the toxicity of the toxin; but if the sample is large and known to be badly contaminated, filtration can be carried out as an additional control. Unfiltered material may also be fed to guinea pigs.

False positive reactions have frequently been mistaken for botulism before typing procedures with antitoxin have been carried out. Nonpathogenic putrefactive organisms can grow in a product of high protein content. When the original product in which these organisms have grown or meat subcultures of these organisms are injected intraperitoneally into mice, the mice may die within 5–30 minutes after injection. Bronfenbrenner, Schlesinger, and Orr (62, 63) found that parenteral introduction of amounts of culture filtrate of *Cl. botulinum* greatly in excess of the minimum lethal dose caused almost immediate death in mice. This result was attributed to the presence in the filtrates of a chemical poison different from botulinum toxin. The poison was not neutralized by antitoxin and was not destroyed by autoclaving in a sealed tube but was lost when autoclaved in an open tube. They identified the volatile substance as ammonia. Also, the statement was made: "It is conceivable that such spoiled foods may be contaminated with common putrefactive bacteria yielding ammonia during their growth and thus may cause death of the test animals."

Other workers have encountered the same phenomenon. Dubovsky and Meyer (64), after examining cultures from soils for *Cl.*

botulinum, make the statement: "Intraperitoneal inoculations, on the other hand, frequently produce shock and sudden death, probably as a result of the various biogenous amines, etc., present in the cultures." Haines (65) encountered the same phenomenon in his examination of some English soils for *Cl. botulinum.* Robinson, Pugh, and Selbie (24) found a convulsant and quickly lethal factor in cultures of anaerobes isolated from whale meat in 23 out of 39 samples. One culture was identified as *Cl. sporogenes.* In the author's experience this reaction has occurred with some extracted food specimens as well as with meat cultures prepared by inoculating beef heart medium with food samples heated at 80° C. for 20 minutes to destroy vegetative cells. When the cultures have been incubated for 5–10 days, the supernatant fluid after centrifugalization may cause sudden death when injected intraperitoneally into mice. Usually a 1–10 dilution of the toxic sample will prove without effect when similarly injected into mice. As final proof of botulinum toxin, reliance must be made on specific neutralization with antitoxin.

Methods of culturing *Cl. botulinum* have been described (66), and the demonstration of *Cl. botulinum* by culture has been resorted to in some outbreaks. One must be very cautious in interpreting such data, since *Cl. botulinum* is ubiquitous and may be a contaminant of any specimen.

The identification of the botulinum toxin is of the greatest value. Sometimes it may be demonstrated in necropsy material from the intestinal tract. It can also be found in serum, as first ascertained by M. Kob (12, 67, 68). Recently, the literature on the demonstration of botulinum toxin in the blood and tissues of patients has been reviewed (69). Obviously, it is important to test the serum of fatal cases for botulinum toxin by the intraperitoneal injection of mice in the laboratory diagnosis of botulism, especially when samples of food are not available. Moreover, in serum samples the gross contamination similar to that encountered in specimens from the bowel is avoided.

The determination of types is established by finding the antitoxin which neutralizes the toxin to be tested. As mentioned previously, the symptoms in the mouse, injected intraperitoneally with the food extract or supernatant fluid from a culture, are the same for all types of botulinum toxin. Serological tests for typing these organisms are not practical, since the groups are heterogeneous (9, 70, 71) and each antitoxin type has several antigenically distinct agglutinative and complement-fixing groups. For this reason, it is time-saving to identify these types simply on a toxigenic basis.

CONTROL OF BOTULISM

The control of botulism requires a knowledge of the responsible bacteria, their habitat in nature, the reason for their growth in preserved foods, and the properties of their toxins.

The organism.—*Clostridium botulinum* is a name applied to a group of rod-shaped, spore-forming, anaerobic bacteria producing exotoxins which may be absorbed from the intestinal tract and which give rise to a common train of symptoms. Five types have been distinguished on the basis of the specific nature of their toxins. These are designated as *Cl. botulinum* or *parabotulinum,* types A, B, C, D, and E. The proteolytic and cultural properties are used by some workers in designating the species as *botulinum* (nonproteolytic) or *parabotulinum* (proteolytic) (72, 73). Animals immunized with a toxin of a specific kind produce antitoxin in their serum for only that type of toxin. The toxin of one type is therefore not neutralized by the antitoxin of a heterologous one. In general, the toxin-antitoxin relationships are constant, although occasionally they vary. For example, a strain of *Cl. botulinum* from Australia resembled *Cl. botulinum* type C, and the toxin produced by this strain could be neutralized by type C antitoxin. The converse, however, was not true, since the antitoxin produced against the Australian toxin would neutralize the Australian toxin but not the toxin produced by type C cultures (74). Human botulism has been reported for types A, B, and E. Types C and D have not been reported as causing human outbreaks of botulism.

Type A and, to a certain extent, type B are proteolytic and digest coagulated egg white, whereas types C, D, and E do not. Gelatin is liquefied by strains of all types. Many of the European type B strains are not proteolytic (75).

In general, the cells of all the types are large, gram-positive rods. The spores are usually subterminal but are terminal in type C. The vegetative cells contain flagella (peritrichate) and are motile under suitable anaerobic conditions.

The biochemical reactions of strains of *Cl. botulinum* vary with reference to certain test substances (Table 8). All strains ferment dextrose, levulose, maltose, and glycerol; but there is considerable variation within the type A and type B strains with reference to the other test substances. Comparatively few strains of types C, D, and E have been tested. Type D strains produce acid only in fermentable test substances; this characteristic separates them from all others.

TABLE 8

FERMENTATION REACTIONS OF VARIOUS TYPES OF
Cl. botulinum AND *Cl. sporogenes*

Type	Dextrose	Levulose	Maltose	Glycerol	Dextrin	Salicin
A............	AG*	AG	AG	AG	AG†	AG†
B............	AG	AG	AG	AG	AG	AG†
C‡...........	AG	AG	AG	AG	AG	O§
D............	A‖	A	A	A	O	O
E............	AG	AG	AG	AG	AG	AG
Cl. sporogenes.	AG	AG	AG	AG	O	O

Type	Galactose	Inositol	Adonitol	Sucrose	Lactose	Raffinose, Insulin, Dulcitol, and Mannitol
A............	O#	O#	O	O	O	O
B............	O	O#	O#	O#	O	O
C‡...........	AG	AG	O	O	O	O
D............	A	A	O	A	A	O
E............	....	AG	AG	AG	....	....
Cl. sporogenes.	O	O	O	O	O	O

* AG = Acid and gas produced.
† Some strains do not ferment.
‡ One C strain from Australia fails to ferment in all tests.
§ O = No acid or gas is produced.
‖ A = Acid only produced.
An occasional strain may ferment.

Clostridium botulinum in the soil.—Since many types of food of both plant and animal origin have been involved in outbreaks of botulism, the natural habitat of *Cl. botulinum* was thought to be soil. A careful study of soils from the United States and from other parts of the world has been made at the Hooper Foundation, University of California (76–82). A less extensive study was made at the University of Chicago under the direction of the late Professor Edwin O.

Jordan, but the results were never reported. Meyer and Dubovsky (78) made an analysis of 1,538 samples of soil, vegetables, feed, and manure collected from every state of the United States except Virginia. They concluded that *Cl. botulinum* is a common soil anaerobe of the western states of the Cordilleran system, is less frequently encountered in the Atlantic states, and is rare in the middle western states, the Great Plains, and the Mississippi Valley. They found that *Cl. botulinum* is more prevalent in virgin soil than in manure or soil collected from animal corrals, pigpens, etc. Vegetables, fruit, and feed are frequently contaminated with the spores of *Cl. botulinum*. String-bean pods and leaves, moldy hay, ensilage, and decayed vegetation may yield a relatively high percentage of positive cultures. Botulinum organisms were not found (77) in land soil of the Aleutian archipelago but were found in moraine, glacier, and mountain soil collected near Lake Louise in the Canadian Rockies. Soil samples from the provinces of Prince Edward Island, Nova Scotia, Quebec, Ontario, and British Columbia have contained *Cl. botulinum*.

Clostridium botulinum type B has been demonstrated in soil and vegetable specimens collected in Belgium, Denmark, England, the Netherlands, and Switzerland (78). It has also been found in soil from the island of Oahu in the Territory of Hawaii and from the provinces of Chilili and Shansi in China (82). Type A has been found in two Hawaiian and one Chinese soil specimen.

From the work reported it is obvious that *Cl. botulinum* is widespread in the soil:

> The soil of the Western States, inclusive of the Great Plains, yield, mainly, *B. botulinus*, Type A, while the Mississippi Valley and Great Lakes region is characterized by a striking predominance of Type B. Similarly prevalent is this latter type in the Atlantic States of Maryland, Delaware, New Jersey, Georgia, and South Carolina, while scattered findings of Type A in Maine, New York, and Pennsylvania indicate the existence of breeding places in virgin forests and mountains. Soils which are subjected to intensive cultivation and fertilization contain, as a rule, *B. botulinus* [= *Cl. botulinum*], Type B [79].

From a total of 2,162 specimens examined (79), 26.8 per cent contained toxic cultures, and 18.2 per cent were typed. This does not mean that nearly three-quarters of the specimens were free of *Cl. botulinum*, because the method of detecting *Cl. botulinum* in soil does not preclude other bacterial species which survive the heat treatment and appear as contaminants. It consists of heating the specimen to destroy many of the less heat-resistant bacteria. The growth of *Cl. botulinum* is demonstrated indirectly by injecting some of the centrifugalized supernatant fluid from the culture into a test animal, either a guinea pig or, more usually, a white mouse. If the animal dies within 4 days, an attempt is made to determine whether or not the toxin is that of *Cl. botulinum* and, if it is, to determine the type. This test is usually done by injecting three mice intraperitoneally with the same dosage that had previously proved fatal (usually 0.5 ml.). Of these three mice, one serves as a control, the second is protected with type A antitoxin, and the third with type B. Other organisms which survive the heat treatment may grow and inhibit the growth of *Cl. botulinum* or destroy botulinum toxin which has been formed. Thus in some soil samples which the author had tested for the presence of *Cl. botulinum*, a toxin was demonstrated which was lethal to mice in 4 days after they had been injected intraperitoneally with 0.5 ml. of the centrifugalized supernatant fluid from the culture. Subsequently, upon attempting to type the toxin, none of the mice receiving the material died. The organism found responsible for destroying the toxin was *Cl. sporogenes* (83). When mixtures of pure cultures of *Cl. sporogenes* and *Cl. botulinum* had been made, *Cl. sporogenes* often overgrew *Cl. botulinum* and subsequently destroyed a portion of the toxin (84). Dubovsky and Meyer (76) observed that "whereas small quantities (10 gm.) of manured soil furnish toxic cultures, 50– or 100–gm. specimens reveal no demonstrable toxin when treated under identical conditions."

These observations make it clear that a negative laboratory test for *Cl. botulinum* does not mean the absence of *Cl. botulinum* in the soil specimen. Furthermore, the demonstration of toxin in over one-fourth of the soils tested indicates that nowhere in nature can soil be considered free from the spores of *Cl. botulinum*. Since the demonstration of the toxin in soil cultures depends in part upon the size of the inoculum (83), botulism may conceivably result from underprocessed food in an area where no *Cl. botulinum* has been demonstrated in soil cultures. Certainly, the amount of soil necessary to contaminate vegetables would be less than the amount of soil used for the detection of the organism in a survey sample.

Effect of moisture and sodium chloride on the growth and toxin production of Clostridium botulinum.—In dehydrated meat (85) experimentally inoculated with the spores of *Cl. botulinum,* type A toxin developed when sufficient water was added to make the moisture content more than 30 per cent. Jensen (86) stated that 3–3.5 per cent salt in cured canned pork and beef meats prevents germination and growth of heavy inocula of spores of aerobic and anaerobic thermophiles.

When cured canned meats containing 3.5 per cent sodium chloride, seeded with *Cl. sporogenes* No. 3679 (N.C.A.) and processed to F_0 1.0, are incubated for 2 years at 99° F., no growth or spoilage takes place (87). A comprehensive test was conducted with spores of *Cl. botulinum* type B No. 213 (88). Thirty thousand to 35,000 spores per gram and 5,000,000 spores per gram were inoculated into two lots of liver sausage (50 per cent moisture) containing 2.78 per cent salt and 3.6 per cent salt, canned in 14-gm. thermal death time cans, and retorted at 235° F. for 4 minutes, and at 2-minute intervals thereafter to 16 minutes. The test lots were incubated at 98° F., and cans were examined for viable spores and toxin at intervals for $1\frac{1}{2}$ years. None of the lots (4–16 minutes) showed growth or toxin formation. Spores were viable up to 1 year. In one test under these conditions, when 30 cans were retorted for 2 minutes only, 2 cans showed growth and toxin in 4 months (88).

A comprehensive test was made with sliced bacon seeded with spores of *Cl. botulinum* type A (89). The slices containing salt (1, 1.25, 1.5, 2, and 2.5 per cent) were placed in vacuum-sealed packages and incubated at 45°, 72°, and 98° F. and were examined for toxin at intervals of from 4 days to 6 months. No toxicity resulted below 72° F. and brine concentrations above 6.5 (1.5 per cent sodium chloride). Identical tests were conducted with vacuum-packed sliced dried beef (10.9–15.7 per cent brine[2]). No toxin developed under these conditions. Country-style cured hams containing 7.7–16.8 per cent brine were also nontoxic when tested in this manner (89). The precise effect of spores of *Cl. botulinum* in meat is detailed elsewhere (90).

Resistance of the spores of Clostridium botulinum to heat.—Outbreaks of botulism occur from eating certain inadequately heat-

2. Brine concentrations are calculated as follows: Canned pork luncheon meat, with 57 per cent moisture and 3.5 per cent sodium chloride = 5.78 per cent brine; liver sausage, with 50 per cent moisture and 3.5 per cent sodium chloride = 6.9 per cent brine; the salt content divided by the sum of moisture and salt and multiplied by 100 = per cent brine.

preserved foods; therefore, the problem of determining the heat resistance of the spores of *Cl. botulinum* is of paramount importance. Heating is a selective process which kills less heat-resistant organisms and permits more heat-resistant types to survive and grow without having to compete with these other forms. Unfortunately, the spores of *Cl. botulinum* are among the more heat-resistant types of microörganisms.

Spores in the dry state are resistant to heat. Old cultures of *Cl. botulinum* type B (91) in brain medium were mixed thoroughly and swabbed on the inside of sterile culture tubes. After drying, they were heated at different temperatures in a Lautenschlager-type gas oven. Tubes were removed at 5-minute intervals, and sterile, freshly boiled dextrose broth was added, after which a sterile paraffin seal was made to keep conditions anaerobic. There was some variation in the heat resistance of five strains tested. At 110° C. the time interval of survival averaged more than 120 minutes. At 140° C. the variation was between 15 and 60 minutes. At 160° and 180° C. the time of survival was between 5 and 15 minutes.

The resistance of *Cl. botulinum* to heat in a liquid substrate appears to differ with the number of spores present. Small numbers—9 or 10 spores—that are present are destroyed within 10 minutes at 100° C., whereas large numbers (92, 93) are more heat-resistant. There is a variation in the different strains. Thus certain strains appear more heat-resistant with few spores present than other strains with large numbers present (80). Esty and Meyer (93) studied the heat resistance of 109 strains of *Cl. botulinum* (78 type A, 30 type B, and 1 nontoxic) from sundry sources. They found that heat resistance varied from 3 to 80 minutes at 105° C. The spores used were from cultures in pea–peptic-digest broth with a pH of 8.0 and were heated in a phosphate solution of pH 7.00–7.12. In some instances the suspensions contained several billion spores. The maximum heat resistance of the spores of *Cl. botulinum* is:

4 min. at 120° C.	. . . .	(248° F.)
10 min. at 115°	. . . .	(239°)
32 min. at 110°	. . . .	(230°)
100 min. at 105°	. . . .	(221°)
330 min. at 100°	. . . .	(212°)

Esty (94) suggested time-temperature relationships for completely destroying all spores of *Cl. botulinum:*

100° C.	360 min.
105°	120 min.
110°	36 min.
115°	12 min.
120°	4 min.

The heat resistance of spores of *Cl. botulinum* type C (72) is
less than types A and B, and these type C spores resist heating to
100° C. for 60 minutes, although not for 90 minutes. Spores of type
D (95), produced in peptic-digest gelatin medium, incubated at
37° C. for 6 days, and diluted to approximately 4,000,000 spores
per milliliter in phosphate solution, survived boiling for 100 minutes
but were destroyed after 120 minutes. Spores of type E (96) resist
temperatures of 80° C. for 10 minutes. Other strains of type E were
tested (97). A suspension of 5,000,000 spores per milliliter in buffer
solution (pH 7.4) failed to show growth after 5 minutes at 100° C.
and after 40 minutes at 80° C. Despite the low heat resistance of
type E, human outbreaks have been reported due to German canned
sprats, Nova Scotia smoked salmon (98), and canned mushroom
sauce (1).

Young spores have been found more heat-resistant than old spores.
When the heat resistance of dried spores was tested in dry heat
(91), a 10-day suspension was found more heat-resistant than a
90-day suspension. In one experiment (93) a strain of *Cl. botulinum*
was grown in pea–peptic-digest broth with and without gelatin and
in neutral brain medium at 37° and 28° C. Tests of resistance were
made from $1\frac{1}{2}$ days through 186 days. Maximum resistance was
obtained in $1\frac{1}{2}$–$3\frac{1}{2}$ days in pea gelatin, $2\frac{1}{4}$ days in pea–peptic-digest,
and 6–16 days in brain medium at 37° C. After these periods, re-
sistance rapidly decreased, although the number of spores present
in the medium remained constant.

Stumbo, Murphy, and Cochran (99) studied high-temperature,
short-time heating of spores of *Cl. botulinum* and, according to their
data, found all thermal death time curves to be essentially straight
lines.

The formation of spores of *Cl. botulinum* is influenced by many
factors, and no methods have been devised for producing uniformly

high yields in laboratory media. Wynne (100) measured the effect of three salts—sodium monosulphate, sodium chloride, and potassium chloride—on the sporulation of type A and found an experimental relationship between concentration of the salts and absolute numbers of spores produced. Blair (101) found that the omission of methionine from a synthetic medium suppressed spore formation of *Cl. botulinum*.

Sodium chloride in concentrations of 8, 10, and 20 per cent solutions greatly decreases the heat resistance of the spores, whereas it is enhanced by solutions from 0.5 to 1.0 per cent concentration. The heat resistance of spores of *Cl. botulinum* in the juices of 17 varieties (93) of canned foods shows variation from less than 10 minutes to 230 minutes at 100° C.

Spores of *Cl. botulinum* types A and B were found to have greater thermal death times when the recovery cultures were incubated at temperatures of 24°–27° C. than when they were incubated at 31° or 37° C. (102).

Ohye and Scott (103) studied the effect of temperature relations on each of 10 strains of *Cl. botulinum* types A and B. Twelve temperatures between 10° and 50° C. were used. Growth proceeded from spore inocula at temperatures from 15° through 42°5 C. but not at 12°5 or 45° C. In the case of type E, Dolman, Chang, Kerr, and Shearer (104) reported that their "VH" strain inoculated into macerated fresh herring gave rise to slight but positive toxin production at 6° C.

Olsen and Scott (105) worked with thirteen strains of *Cl. botulinum* types A and B and found that the detection and enumeration of spores surviving lethal heating became increasingly difficult as the period of heating was increased, as the surviving spores became more sensitive to inhibitors in the medium. These inhibitory substances were present in all media tested, and their effects were counteracted under a wide range of conditions by the incorporation of approximately 0.1 per cent starch. However, the starch did not affect the estimates of unheated spores. Olsen and Scott (105) accounted for the effects of starch as a feature of the amylose portion of the undegraded starch molecule, which, like charcoal or serum albumin, acts by adsorbing inhibitors from the medium.

Factors affecting the heat resistance of spores have been studied by Sugiyama (106, 107). He observed that spores of *Cl. botulinum* formed at 37° C. are of higher heat resistance than those developed at 41°, 29°, or 24° C. The addition of Ca^{++} and Mg^{++} to the spore-suspending menstruum was found to reduce the heat tolerance of the spores. The sodium chloride concentration of the sporulating medium had no significant effect on the heat resistance of the spores. Below a certain concentration, the lower the Fe^{++} and Ca^{++} concentration of the sporulating medium, the lower the thermostability of the spores. The heat resistance of spores suspended in different concentrations of sucrose was found to increase with the concentration of sucrose. Spores suspended in 50 per cent sucrose increase almost immediately in heat resistance, and this increase remains high for hours. Fatty acids in the sporulating medium were found to influence the heat tolerance of the spores. In general, the longer the fatty-acid chain, the greater the increase in thermal tolerance. In order not to suppress germination, Sugiyama found it necessary to remove the excess fatty-acid salts from the spore suspension.

There may be a marked delay in the germination of spores of *Cl. botulinum* after they have been heated. Dickson and his co-workers (108) observed that some tubes of medium containing small numbers of heated spores would remain apparently sterile for weeks or months after others had shown growth but would eventually exhibit vigorous growth with toxin formation. Appearance of growth after 72 months has been reported (109).

The problem of heat penetration is extremely important when dealing with foods. In large gallon containers, it is difficult to heat certain products so that the center of the cans will contain no viable *Cl. botulinum* without impairing the product. This problem is well understood by the commercial canner. For example, each specific food item is tested in the laboratory before processing times and temperatures are recommended. Of these various tests (110), the concern is with the rate of heat penetration in different containers under laboratory and factory conditions.

The foregoing studies on the heat resistance of the spores of *Cl. botulinum* should convince everyone that home canning by the cold-pack method, which is still widely used in the United States, is extremely dangerous. It is to be hoped, however, that the advice constantly given by the schools, the press, and the radio will have effect, so that the pressure-cooker method will be used for canning instead of the cold-pack method.

Botulism may be prevented if sufficient care is given to home canning. It is important that fresh, firm fruits and vegetables are thoroughly washed, cleaned, and canned as soon as possible after having been picked or gathered. Nonacid foods, such as vegetables, meat, poultry, or fish, should be processed in a pressure cooker for a specific period of time (111) with an accurate gauge or ther-mometer. Where canning is done by any other method, the food should be reboiled for 15 minutes (actual boiling time) before tast-ing or eating. A canned food with a disagreeable odor or showing gas pressure should not be tasted under any circumstances. Spoiled food of this type should be treated by adding several spoonfuls of lye to the can or jar; the can should then be kept for not less than 24 hours and then should be buried. A glass container should be carefully soaked in a hot lye solution after the spoiled food has been destroyed.

Other factors affecting the growth of Clostridium botulinum.— The germination of spores of *Cl. botulinum* requires a higher tem-perature of incubation than growth and multiplication alone. Growth and toxin production occurs within a few days at 20° C., when either vegetative cells or spores are inoculated. When vegetative cells are inoculated into suitable media held at 15° C., toxin is pro-duced, but heat-detoxified spores rarely produce toxin at this tem-perature. Tanner and Oglesby (112) observed that foods stored at room temperature or under slight refrigeration may become danger-ous rapidly, but they will remain safe for a considerable length of time at less than 10° C. *Clostridium botulinum* may sometimes de-velop and produce toxin in frozen foods which have been allowed to thaw and have been stored at temperatures of 10° C. or higher. However, frozen foods, if properly handled and kept frozen until used, are probably as safe and satisfactory as fresh foods (113).

Antibiotics have been studied with reference to their effect on spore germination. Penicillin was found by Wynne (100) to have no effect on the germination of spores of *Cl. botulinum*, and Collier and Wynne (114) reported no effect on germination of the spores of *Cl. botulinum* with streptomycin. In the case of subtilin, Andersen (115) observed that 0.4 p.p.m. prevented as many as 517 spores of

Cl. botulinum type A from producing colonies in pork-infusion agar. One p.p.m. subtilin allowed 253 out of 800,000 spores to produce colonies. Cameron and Bohrer (116) inoculated canned peas containing 20 p.p.m. subtilin with 1,000 and 500,000 spores per can, after which the cans were heated to 93° C. Botulinum spoilage occurred at both levels of inoculum in the case of type A and at only the higher level of inoculum in the case of type B. Williams and Fleming (117) observed a difference among individual strains of *Cl. botulinum* types A and B in sensitivity to subtilin in culture medium, although there is no difference that distinguishes the types. The time required for appearance of growth from spores increased with an enlargement in subtilin content combined with large inocula. These studies also indicated that subtilin was not sporocidal but sporostatic instead.

The effect of fatty acids on the germination of spores has been studied. Foster and Wynne (118) found that oleic, linoleic, and linolenic acids inhibited germination of spores of *Cl. botulinum*. Roth and Halvorson (119) showed that these fatty acids and their methyl esters were inhibitory only when rancid. Benzoyl peroxide inhibited in the same order of magnitude as rancid, unsaturated fatty acids. Catalase only partially reversed the inhibition caused by the rancid fatty acids.

Wynne and Foster (120) noted that the germination of spores of *Cl. botulinum* was affected by minute amounts of substances in the general category of impurities. Such impurities occur in all organic media and possibly in tap water. When soluble starch was incorporated into the media used for testing the germination of spores, more uniform results occurred between replicate tube counts of a given dilution. The starch was thought to have an adsorption effect on the impurities. The germination process of spores of one strain of *Cl. botulinum*, 62A, was found to be logarithmic (121). When exposed to air the lag period in germination varied inversely with the logarithm of the number of spores per milliliter in the inoculum.

Beets and carrots canned in plain unlacquered cans were found not to support the growth of either type A or type B experimentally inoculated into the cans (122). In similar experiments with lacquered cans, growth and toxin production occurred. The addition of a soluble tin citrate complex to each vegetable produced inhibition of growth in both lacquered cans and test tubes. Concentrations of tin required to prevent growth were approximately 150 p.p.m. in beets and 30–60 p.p.m. in carrots. This study was extended to include nine additional vegetables (123). Inhibition of growth, at 20°, 30°, and 37° C., for periods up to 6 months was observed in plain cans of French-style beans (cut green beans), silver beets (Swiss chard), and parsnips, beets, and carrots. No inhibition was observed in plain cans of asparagus, cabbage, cauliflower, peas, potatoes, and white turnips. Inhibition of growth in plain cans was bacteriostatic and was associated with concentrations of dissolved tin which exceeded the values for lacquered cans. The concentration of tin in solution found necessary to prevent growth differed considerably between vegetables and was positively correlated with reported protein contents. Under no circumstances should dissolved tin in a product be relied upon to replace safe processing of canned goods.

PATHOGENICITY OF *Clostridium Botulinum*

Outbreaks of human botulism are caused principally by the exotoxins of types A and B. A few outbreaks have been caused by the exotoxins of type E. Outbreaks of animal botulism are caused by exotoxins of *Cl. botulinum* types C and D.

Type D, isolated from toxic carrion in South Africa, produces *lamziekte*, a fatal cattle disease in Bechuanaland, Orange Free State, and in the northwest portion of the Cape Province. The disease *lamziekte* was renamed "parabotulinum" when the organism isolated from the specimens in question by Theiler and his associates (124) was called *Clostridium parabotulinum bovis*. In the same year, Theiler and Robinson (125, 126) described an organism of the *parabotulinum* group which was isolated from the carcass of a dead rat found in a haystack near a stable. This organism was supposedly connected with spinal paralysis of mules or equine parabotulism. The biochemical reactions of type D are listed in Table 8. Small doses of toxin appear to be fatal to ruminants *per os*, particularly goats and cattle, but not to laboratory rodents and apes (95). In fact, the fatal feeding dose is at least two hundred to three thousand times that of the inoculating dose. The susceptibility of the guinea pig, mouse, and rabbit to subcutaneous injections of type D toxin is the same as for types A, B, and C. When injected subcutaneously into a chicken, 100,000 guinea-pig M.L.D. of the type D toxin are without effect. The chicken is resistant to subcutaneous injection of *Cl. botulinum* type B. Again, the monkey is resistant to type D toxin given orally in doses of 40,000 and 200,000 guinea-pig M.L.D. Whether man is susceptible to type D toxin *per os* is not known; but, as no human cases have been reported, man may possibly be as resistant as the monkey.

Type E produces a toxin of varying potency, depending upon the strain. Dolman *et al.* (104) described 6 outbreaks in Canada, involving 38 persons and 22 deaths. *Clostridium botulinum* type E has been found principally in canned fish. In Japan, botulism cases were not reported until June, 1951, when an outbreak occurred in Hokkaido. Of 7 persons affected, 4 died within 3 days after eating "izushi," a Japanese home-prepared food from rice, fish, and vegetables eaten only in northern Japan. During the period from June, 1951, to August, 1954, 6 outbreaks involving 25 cases with 10 deaths occurred, and type E was isolated in all outbreaks (127, 128). Prévot and Huet (129) isolated a type E strain from the intestinal tract of a perch from which a toxin with an M.L.D. of 0.01 ml. for mice (intraperitoneal) was prepared. Gunnison, Cummings, and Meyer (97) worked with a strain of such potency that a subcutaneous injection of 0.02 ml. is an M.L.D. for a 350-gm. guinea pig. Hazen (130) observed characteristic symptoms of botulism following the subcutaneous injection of the toxin into guinea pigs, mice, rabbits, and kittens. He found the toxins produced by 2 different strains of *Cl. botulinum* type E, although reciprocally neutralized by their antitoxins, to differ in their effect when subcutaneously injected into White Leghorn chickens. Slocum, Welch, and Hunter (14) attempted to determine the M.L.D. of two strains of type E in guinea pigs. The M.L.D. was found for one strain, but the other strain was apparently atoxic, since several hundred times the dose for the toxic strain failed to produce death or symptoms of botulism in guinea pigs.

The temperature for growth of one strain of *Cl. botulinum* type E was tested in beef heart medium stored at $10°$, $12°8$, and $15°5$ C., $(50°$, $55°$, and $60°$ F.) (131). Tubes of this medium which had been boiled and cooled were inoculated with spores of a culture[3] isolated from herring and sealed with sterile vaseline. To destroy the toxin, the spore suspension was heated at 80° C. for 10 minutes before inoculation. There were 1,400 viable spores per milliliter of beef heart medium immediately after inoculation. At 15°5 C., growth and toxin production occurred in 2 weeks, but not in 1 week. At 12°8 C. there was good growth and toxin production after 4 weeks but not in 2 weeks. No growth or toxin was observed after 4, 6, 8, 12, 16, or 26 weeks at 10° C.

In comparison with type E, growth and toxin production of types A and B occurred after 1 week at 15°5 C. However, the same mixture of spores of types A and B required 6 weeks before toxin could be found in the undiluted culture at 12°8 C. At subsequent intervals of 8, 12, 16, and 26 weeks no more toxin was produced, since it was not detected in 1:10 dilutions tested at these intervals. No growth occurred at these intervals at 10° C.

Clostridium botulinum type C has not been reported as being responsible for human botulism. Bengtson (132) first isolated type C from fly larvae and showed that the toxin was not neutralized by antitoxin for types A and B. Kalmbach (133) made a study of so-called "duck sickness," which is widespread in nature. In 1910 untold thousands of waterfowl died in the marshes around Great Salt Lake, Utah, and the years following saw a recurrence of the sickness but to a lesser degree. Nearly 50,000 ducks were buried at the mouth of Bear River, Utah, from September 7 to September 26, 1913. Kalmbach reproduced the disease in ducks by feeding body tissues, which had been kept at a temperature of 85° F. for 5 or more days, from birds dead from duck sickness. Giltner and Couch (134) isolated *Cl. botulinum* type C from mud and water from an infected area in Tule Lake, California, while an outbreak was at its height. Type C has been cultured from the tissues of wild mallards, pintails, and ring-billed gulls which died while afflicted with the disease.

Duck sickness has been reported in the Province of Alberta, Canada, about 45 miles east of the city of Calgary and 130 miles north of the Montana border (135). In the summer of 1940 several hundred wild ducks died in a bird sanctuary in Jackson Park, Chi-

3. Obtained from Dr. C. E. Dolman, Vancouver, British Columbia.

cago; yet no evidence of the disease was found in Lincoln Park, some 10 miles north. Maggots and livers taken from the dead ducks were studied by Dr. Ellen Davison.[4] The maggots and liver were ground separately in sterile mortars with sterile sand and saline solution. The samples were centrifugalized to eliminate the gross particles and then filtered through Berkefeld filters. Toxin was demonstrated in the liver and in the filtrate of the maggot extract. This toxin was neutralized by *Cl. botulinum* type C antitoxin. Toxicity tests were made by inoculating white mice subcutaneously and making appropriate toxin controls. Duck sickness occurs during the hot months of the year in stagnant waters but apparently not in large bodies of water. The toxin evidently continues to be formed after the death of the animal and thereby contributes to the toxicity of the water.

There are many problems regarding type C botulism which are unsolved. Much needs to be learned regarding the behavior of the organism in nature. The abundance of the organisms in the tissues after death suggests either an ante mortem spread of the organism or a rapid post mortem invasion of the tissues, with a predominance over other naturally occurring microörganisms. Gunnison and Meyer (136) found that the rhesus monkey is resistant to the toxin of types C and D when they are given orally. It is possible that if more potent toxin had been used by these investigators, the monkeys would have been found susceptible. Meat cultures of types C and E fed to *Macaca mulatta* by Wagenaar *et al.* (57) readily caused botulism.

The problem arises as to the danger of botulism from the ingestion of large numbers of organisms. Suppose, for example, that a preserved food contains a large number of the incriminating organisms and that in its preparation for consumption it is sufficiently heated to destroy the toxin and not the spores. Could botulism occur? Coleman and Meyer (137) and Starin and Dack (138) have answered this question negatively. It is their conclusion that the danger of botulism from toxin-free spores could follow only after the ingestion of an enormous number of spores.

Since the spores of *Cl. botulinum* are present in the soil and are widespread in nature, they are undoubtedly swallowed in small numbers with dust, dirt, uncooked fresh fruits, and vegetables. Ex-

4. University of Chicago.

perience, however, has shown that botulism does not occur in this manner. Furthermore, if small numbers of *Cl. botulinum* organisms should grow in the intestinal tract and produce minute amounts of toxin, we should expect to find small amounts of antitoxin in the serum of animals. This is apparently not the case. The conclusion, therefore, can be drawn that the toxin of *Cl. botulinum* must be ingested to produce botulism.

TOXIN OF *Clostridium botulinum*

The toxin of *Cl. botulinum* is a true exotoxin, which gives rise to characteristic symptoms when injected into animals. The specific types produce specific antitoxins in the serum of immunized animals. The one irregularity, as mentioned before, is the observation of Pfenninger (74) that an Australian strain from Dr. Seddon produces a toxin which is neutralized by type C antitoxin but that the antitoxin prepared for the Australian strain does not neutralize the toxin of American strains of type C.

As indicated in the beginning of the chapter, various kinds of food have been involved in outbreaks of botulism. However, many of these foods are poor media for good growth and toxin production. If they were good media, it is likely that signs of spoilage would be more evident, and they would be discarded and not eaten. Growth and toxin of *Cl. botulinum* have been produced in chemically defined media (139), but, in general, toxin of low potency occurs under these circumstances. Very potent type A toxin has been produced in media containing powdered milk, casein, glucose, and clarified corn-steep liquor (140). Type A toxin has been crystallized from filtrates of cultures using this medium.

The toxin of *Cl. botulinum* type A was obtained in crystalline form by two groups of workers at approximately the same time (141, 142). Type A toxin behaves like a globulin with an isoelectric point of pH 5.6 and a total nitrogen of 14.1–14.3 per cent. The toxin crystallized readily in 0.10–0.30 saturated ammonium sulphate at 4° C., forming small needle-like crystals. An LD_{50} for the 20-gm. white mouse contains 4.5×10^{-9} mg. of nitrogen, and there are about 32,000,000,000 intraperitoneal LD_{50} per gram of dry toxin (143). The molecular weight based on studies of diffusion, apparent specific volume, and viscosity performed on crystalline materials was found to be 1,130,000 (144). By electrophoretic sedimentation and diffusion characteristics of the crystalline protein made by another group of workers (145), the molecular weight was calculated to be 900,000.

Wagman and Bateman (146) measured the sedimentation rate and diffusion constant of two specimens of type A botulinum toxin at pH 3.8–4.4, indicating a molecular weight of about 940,000 and an axial ratio of 17.5. The molecular weight of type B toxin, determined similarly at pH 3.0, was about 500,000. At pH 7.5 about 14 per cent of the material in solution of type A toxin appeared as a second component, of sedimentation constant 7. This component was separated in the ultracentrifuge. Subsequently, Wagman and Bateman (147) measured sedimentation and diffusion constants of a specimen of "dissociated toxin" separated in the ultracentrifuge and found a value of 71,000 for the molecular weight and 3.4 for the axial ratio. The toxicity of this low-molecular-weight product formed at pH 7.5 is at least as great, per milligram protein nitrogen, as the parent-substance. The flocculation titer is the same as the parent-substance, but the hemagglutinin titer is essentially zero. The nonhemagglutinating polydisperse "dissociated toxin" of molecular weight around 70,000 is identified tentatively with the ultimate toxic unit of type A botulinum toxin. In a subsequent study, Wagman (148) placed some type A toxin in a phosphate buffer (at pH 7.5 and ionic strength 1.0) after first isolating from it, by differential centrifugation, some of the low-molecular-weight material formed in more dilute phosphate (ionic strength 0.13 at the same pH), leaving only the slowly sedimenting fraction in solution. The low-molecular-weight fraction, separated at ionic strength 1.0, possessed a specific toxicity two to three times that of the original sample and differed in this and other properties from the low-molecular-weight material separated at ionic strength 0.13. From these and other data on toxicity, hemagglutinating activity, and sedimentation behavior of the several fractions, Wagman has constructed a hypothetical structure for the type A toxin particle of molecular weight 10^6 which consists of an assembly of toxic and inert subunits in association with one or more hemagglutinin units.

The elemental and amino acid composition of crystalline *Cl. botu-*

linum type A toxin has been determined (149). The chemical entities which were found are shown in the accompanying tabulation.

	Per Cent		Per Cent
Lysine	7.74	Asparagine	20.10
Histidine	1.03	Serine	4.36
Arginine	4.63	Threonine	8.49
Tyrosine	13.50	Cysteine	0.268
Phenylalanine	1.17	Half-cystine	0.534
Tryptophan	1.86	Methionine	1.06
Valine	5.29	Proline	2.60
Leucine	10.30	Glycine	1.38
Isoleucine	11.94	Alanine	3.92
Glutamic acid	15.57		

The authors were unable to explain the extreme toxicity of the protein on the basis of their analytical data. Lamanna (150) found that crystalline type A toxin possessed a hemagglutinating activity which was found by Lamanna and Lowenthal (151) to be separate from the toxin. The hemagglutinin was removed by agglutinin-absorption techniques, leaving only one component, the toxin.

Type B toxin has been purified (152) by methods involving acid precipitations and working with the toxin on the acid side of its isoelectric zone. The purified toxin was not crystalline and appeared to be a slightly colored, simple protein, soluble in water on the acid side of the isoelectric range, and relatively insoluble on the alkaline side and within the isoelectric range. Slight additions of salt did not increase the solubility of the purified toxin. The molecular size, estimated with a sintered-glass membrane diffusion apparatus, was about 60,000 in contrast to the much higher figure for the crystalline type A toxin (900,000–1,200,000). Serologically, chemically, and physically the purified type B toxin differs from type A crystalline toxin. Its toxicity per milligram of nitrogen is only slightly less than that of type A, but on a molar basis it would appear to be ten times less potent. The guinea pig is approximately three times more susceptible to the toxin than the white mouse when the toxin is injected intraperitoneally.

Nigg *et al.* (153) prepared toxoids from types A and B botulinum toxin. When these toxoids were tested in animals (154), a marked difference was found in the antigenic response of mice to fluid and to alum-precipitated botulinum toxoid. One dose of fluid toxoid induced little immunity in mice, whereas immunity was obtained with a single dose of alum-precipitated toxoid. Guinea pigs developed immunity following single-dose injections of fluid and of alum-precipitated botulinum toxoid. Type A botulinum toxoid has been prepared from crystalline toxin by the addition of formaldehyde (155). One preparation, consisting of one component electrophoretically, immunized mice in a dose containing 0.01γ of toxoid nitrogen and was twenty-four hundred times more active antigenically than crude toxoid on the basis of nitrogen content.

Fluid and alum-precipitated type A and B botulinum toxoids were used to immunize a man (156). Excellent results were obtained; thus the method is practical in protecting laboratory personnel working with these toxins against accidents where the toxin may gain entrance into the body.

There is a closer relationship between *Cl. botulinum* types C and D than that which exists among types A, B, and C. The lethal toxin and hemagglutinins in antiserum of types C and D are not identical. Lamanna (157) found that hemagglutination of red cells by supernatants of *Cl. botulinum* type C cultures was specific, since the reaction could be inhibited by antiserum to type C and not by antisera to types A and B. Sterne (158) studied the relationship between types C and D and found that hemagglutination of sheep cells by type D filtrate was inhibited by antisera to both types C and D, although the specific type C antiserum contained no demonstrable antibody to the toxin of type D. However, it is not unusual for high-titer type C antisera to contain a small amount of antibody to type D toxin, and vice versa.

Wentzel, Sterne, and Polson (159) grew cultures of *Cl. botulinum* type D in intussuscepted cellophane tubes. They found that the major portion of the toxin could be precipitated by using a 40 per cent saturation with ammonium sulphate. By subsequent redissolving and precipitating with 25 and 30 per cent saturation of ammonium sulphate at pH 5.8, a final toxin was obtained which was dialyzed and found to be electrophoretically homogeneous. Diffusion measurements indicated that the material was polydisperse and that the major part diffused at a rate consistent with an average molecular weight of about a million.

Toxicity was measured by injecting 20-gm. white mice with

appropriate dilutions, with eight mice for each dilution. When the toxin was diluted in 0.2 per cent gelatin in phosphate buffer at pH 6.2, the very high toxicity of 4×10^{12} M.L.D./mg protein nitrogen was obtained, which appeared to be about twenty thousand times as toxic for the mouse as pure type A toxin.

According to Therber *et al.* (160) an estimated 50,000 head of cattle die yearly from eating carrion infected with type C and D botulinum toxins. In Australia, according to Bennetts and Hall (161), heavy losses have occurred due to type C toxin. Although in Australia toxoids have been used for immunizing animals to type C and in South Africa to types C and D, Sterne and Wentzel (162) have prepared potent botulinum toxin, types C and D, by using in-tussuscepted cellophane tubing immersed in nutrient broth. The "dialyzate" toxin is fifty to a hundred times as potent as toxins prepared in the conventional manner. They have prepared formol-toxoids from these "dialyzate" toxins which are up to eight thousand times as efficient in eliciting immunity response. A dose that will provoke a high antibody titer in the serum of cattle may contain as little as 0.001 mg. protein nitrogen. Boroff and Cabeen (163) have described an atoxic variant of *Cl. botulinum* type C, which, injected intravenously into rabbits, induced the formation of protective and flocculating antibodies active against the toxic form.

— *Heat resistance of botulinum toxin.*—In contrast to the heat resistance of the spores, the toxins are susceptible to heat. Data on the heat resistance of the type A toxin are summarized by Meyer (9). At 80° C. the toxin is destroyed in from 30 seconds to 6 minutes; at 72° C. in from 2 to 18 minutes; and at 65° C. within 10–85 minutes. The toxin of certain strains of type B has been found to require 15 minutes at 80° C. for destruction, whereas the toxin of type C strains appears to require more heat, i.e., 30 minutes at 80° C. (Bengtson), 6–8 minutes at 80° C. (Schoenholz and Meyer), and 15 minutes at 80° C. (Seddon).

Scott and Stewart (164) studied the rate of destruction of type A and B toxins in a variety of canned vegetables. For type A toxin, they found that destruction at 80° C. proceeds at least a hundred times as rapidly as at 70° C. and the stability of the toxin was greatest at pH 5.0. Vegetable liquors contained dissolved substances which helped to protect the toxin against destruction with heat. The heat stability of the toxin varied with the product. In any one vegetable the rate of destruction was found to be the same as for toxin produced by other type A strains. Type B toxin was destroyed more readily than type A in all products. Vegetable liquors protected the toxin, but the effect of pH was not as great as with type A toxin.

Scott (165) in a further study reported that the heat stability of type A toxin in canned vegetables is due to the various ionized substances dissolved in them. In canned cabbage, salts of common inorganic and organic acids are sufficient to explain the observed protection, but in canned carrots other substances are involved. At pH 5.0 protection is afforded by both cations and anions, although some substances are more effective than others at low concentrations. The protective effects of several different ions were found to be additive, and the toxin was most stable in mixtures of high ionic strength. Therefore, the ionic environment of the toxin must be known if the time and temperature conditions necessary for the destruction of a given amount of toxin are to be specified.

From these data it can be seen that toxins are not destroyed when foods are merely warmed. Thus, before consumption, food should be boiled and thoroughly mixed during the boiling process so that a temperature is reached that will destroy the toxin throughout the preparation.

REFERENCES

1. GEIGER, J. C. J.A.M.A., **117**:22, 1941.
2. DAUER, C. C. Pub. Health Rep., **67**:1089–95, 1951.
3. MEYER, K. F. New England J. Med., **249**:765–73, 804–12, 843–52, 1953.
4. DAUER, C. C., and SYLVESTER, GRANVILLE. Pub. Health Rep., **69**: 538–46, 1954.
5. DAUER, C. C. Pub. Health Rep., **68**:696–702, 1953.
6. MEYER, K. F., and EDDIE, B. Fifty years of botulism in U.S. and Canada, July, 1950. Mimeographed report from George Williams Hooper Foundation, University of California.
7. DICKSON, ERNEST C. Monogr. Rockefeller Inst. M. Res., No. 8, 1918.
8. ERMENGEM, E. VAN. Rev. d'hyg. **18**:1–61, 1896.
9. MEYER, K. F. Handb. d. path. Mikroorg., **4**:1269–1364, 1928.
10. GEIGER, J. C., DICKSON, E. C., and MEYER, K. F. Pub. Health Bull. 127, 1922.
11. ZLATOGOROFF, S. I., and SOLOVIEV, M. N. J.A.M.A., **88**:2024–26, 1927.
12. KOSER, STEWART A., and REITER, DOROTHY O. J. Prevent. Med., **3**: 499–504, 1929.

13. WAGENAAR, R. O., and DACK, G. M. Food Res., **19**:521–29, 1954.
14. SLOCUM, G. G., WELCH, HENRY, and HUNTER, ALBERT C. Food Res., **6**:179–87, 1941.
15. HALL, IVAN C. Am. J. Hyg., **17**:235–51, 1933.
16. ———. Food Res., **1**:171–98, 1936.
17. HUNTER, CHARLES A., WEISS, JAMES E., and OLSON, C. L. Journal-Lancet, **60**:67–69, 1940.
18. INGRAM, M., and ROBINSON, R. H. M. Proc. Soc. Appl. Bact., **14**:73–84, 1951.
19. TOWNSEND, CHARLES T., YEE, LOIS, and MERCER, WALTER A. Food Res., **19**:536–42, 1954.
20. KADAVY, JOAN L., and DACK, G. M. Food Res., **16**:328–37, 1951.
21. INGRAM, M., and ROBINSON, R. H. M. Proc. Soc. Appl. Bact., **14**:62–72, 1951.
22. WAGENAAR, R. O., and DACK, G. M. Food Res., **20**:144–48, 1955.
23. SEGALOVE, MILTON, and DACK, G. M. Food Res., **16**:118–25, 1951.
24. ROBINSON, R. H. M., PUGH, A. M., and SELBIE, F. R. J. Hyg., **47**:236–43, 1949.
25. STEINKE, P. K. W., and FOSTER, E. M. Food Res., **16**:477–84, 1951.
26. WAGENAAR, R. O., and DACK, G. M. Two abstracts from J. Dairy Sc., **36**:563–64, 1953, and **37**:640, 1954.
27. ALLEN, ROBERT W., and ECKLUND, A. WALTER. J.A.M.A., **99**:557–59, 1932.
28. CARY, W. E. Personal communication.
29. DACK, GAIL M., and WOOD, WILLARD L. J. Infect. Dis., **42**:209–12, 1928.
30. Personal communication from Dr. O. C. Woolpert, who observed the cases.
31. VELIKANOV, I. M., and KOLESNIKOVA, M. K. Klin. med., **12**:1807–52, 1934; abstr., J.A.M.A., **104**:1050, 1935.
32. WATSON, W. E. Northwest Med., **38**:382–87, 1939.
33. CAPRIO, FRANK S. J.A.M.A., **106**:687–89, 1936.
34. TUCKER, C. B., and SWANSON, HOMER. Pub. Health Rep., **54**:1556–60, 1939.
35. ORTON, HENRY B. Ann. Otol., Rhin. & Laryng., **60**:485–95, 1951.
36. DACK, G. M., and HOSKINS, DOROTHY. J. Infect. Dis., **71**:260–63, 1942.
37. HAEREM, SARAH, DACK, G. M., and DRAGSTEDT, LESTER R. Surgery, **3**:339–50, 1938.
38. DACK, G. M., and GIBBARD, J. J. Infect. Dis., **39**:173–80, 1926.
39. DICKSON, ERNEST C., and SHEVKY, RICHARD. J. Exper. Med., **37**:711–31, 1923.
40. ———. *Ibid.*, **38**:327–46, 1923.
41. EDMUNDS, CHARLES W., and LONG, PERRIN H. J.A.M.A., **81**:542–47, 1923.
42. BISHOP, GEORGE H., and BRONFENBRENNER, JACQUES J. Am. J. Physiol., **117**:393–404, 1936.
43. GUYTON, ARTHUR C., and MacDONALD, MARSHALL A. Arch. Neurol. & Psychiat., **57**:578–92, 1947, with additions.

44. Masland, R. L., and Gammon, G. D. J. Pharmacol. & Exper. Therap., **97**:499–506, 1949.
45. Torda, Clara, and Wolff, Harold G. J. Pharmacol. & Exper. Therap., **89**:320–24, 1947.
46. Burgen, A. S. V., Dickens, F., and Zatman, L. J. J. Physiol. (London), **109**:10–24, 1949.
47. Ambache, N. Brit. J. Pharmacol., **6**:51–67, 1951.
48. ———. J. Physiol. (London), **113**:1–17, 1951.
49. ———. *Ibid.*, **116**:9, 1952.
50. Stover, J. H., Jr., Fingerman, M., and Forester, R. H. Proc. Soc. Exper. Biol. & Med., **84**:146–47, 1953.
51. Brooks, Vernon B. Science, **117**:334–35, 1953.
52. Davies, Joan R., Morgan, R. S., Wright, E. A., and Wright, G. P. J. Physiol. (London), **120**:618–23, 1953.
53. Moll, T., and Brandly, C. A. Am. J. Vet. Res., **12**:355–63, 1951.
54. Quortrup, E. R., and Holt, A. L. J. Am. Vet. M. A., **97**:167–68, 1940.
55. Dinter, Z., and Kull, K. E. Nord. vet. med., **3**:297–311, 1951.
56. Kull, K. E. von, and Moberg, K. Nord. vet. med., **4**:771–79, 1952.
57. Wagenaar, R. O., Dack, G. M., and Mayer, D. P. Am. J. Vet. Res., **14**:479–83, 1953.
58. Cartwright, T. E., and Lauffer, Max A. Proc. Soc. Exper. Biol. & Med., **81**:508–11, 1952.
59. Graham, Robert, and Schwarze, Herman. J.A.M.A., **76**:1743–44, 1921.
60. Leighton, G. Botulism, p. 205. London: W. Collins Sons & Co., Ltd., 1923.
61. Schoenholz, P., Esty, J. R., and Meyer, K. F. J. Infect. Dis., **33**: 289–327, 1923.
62. Bronfenbrenner, J., Schlesinger, M. J., and Orr, P. F. Proc. Soc. Exper. Biol. & Med., **18**:181–82, 1921.
63. ———. J. Exper. Med., **40**:81–89, 1924.
64. Dubovsky, Bertha J., and Meyer, K. F. J. Infect. Dis., **31**:523, 1922.
65. Haines, R. B. J. Hyg., **42**:324, 1942.
66. Dack, Gail M. Am. J. Pub. Health, **16**:744–45, 1926.
67. Kob, M. Med. Klin., **1**:84–86, 1904–5.
68. Bengtson, I. A. Pub. Health Rep., **36**:1665–71, 1921.
69. Schneider, Harry J., and Fisk, Roy. J.A.M.A., **113**:2299–2300, 1939.
70. Starin, William A., and Dack, Gail M. J. Infect. Dis., **33**:169–83, 1923.
71. ———. *Ibid.*, **34**:137–47, 1924.
72. Bengtson, I. A. Hyg. Lab. Bull. 136, 1924.
73. Gunnison, J. B., and Meyer, K. F. J. Infect. Dis., **45**:119–34, 1929.
74. Pfenninger, W. J. Infect. Dis., **35**:346, 1924.
75. Meyer, K. F. Modern medical therapy in general practice, p. 1176. Baltimore: Williams & Wilkins Co., 1940.

76. Dubovsky, Bertha J., and Meyer, K. F. J. Infect. Dis., **31**:501–40, 1922.
77. ———. *Ibid.*, pp. 595–99.
78. Meyer, K. F., and Dubovsky, Bertha J. J. Infect. Dis., **31**:541–55, 1922.
79. ———. *Ibid.*, pp. 559–94.
80. ———. *Ibid.*, pp. 600–609.
81. Coleman, George E. J. Infect. Dis., **31**:556–58, 1922.
82. Schoenholz, P., and Meyer, K. F. J. Infect. Dis., **31**:610–13, 1922.
83. Jordan, Edwin O., and Dack, Gail M. J. Infect. Dis., **35**:576–80, 1924.
84. Dack, G. M. J. Infect. Dis., **38**:165–73, 1926.
85. U.S. Dept. Agr., Circ. No. 706, p. 21, August, 1944.
86. Jensen, L. B. Microbiology of meats, pp. 311–13. 2d ed. Champaign, Ill.: Garrard Press, 1945.
87. ———. Bact. Rev., **8**:161–88, 1944.
88. ———. Unpublished material, in collaboration with Dr. R. W. Pilcher and Dr. Evan Wheaton. Maywood, Ill., American Can Co.
89. ———. Unpublished material, in collaboration with Dr. G. M. Dack, Dr. E. Hemmens, and Joan Kadavy, at the University of Chicago.
90. ———. Microbiology of meats. 3d ed. Champaign, Ill.: Garrard Press, 1954.
91. Tanner, Fred W., and Dack, Gail M. J. Infect. Dis., **31**:92–100, 1922.
92. Starin, William A. J. Infect. Dis., **38**:101–5, 1926.
93. Esty, J. R., and Meyer, K. F. J. Infect. Dis., **31**:650–63, 1922.
94. Esty, J. Russell. Am. J. Pub. Health, **13**:108–13, 1923.
95. Meyer, K. F., and Gunnison, J. B. J. Infect. Dis., **49**:106–18, 1929.
96. Hazen, E. L. J. Infect. Dis., **60**:259–64, 1937.
97. Gunnison, J. B., Cummings, J. R., and Meyer, K. F. Proc. Soc. Exper. Biol. & Med., **35**:278–80, 1936.
98. Mackenzie, G. M. Clin. misc., Mary Imogene Bassett Hosp., Cooperstown, N.Y., **1**:53, 1934.
99. Stumbo, C. R., Murphy, J. R., and Cochran, Jeanne. Food Technol., **4**:321–26, 1950.
100. Wynne, E. Staten. Bact. Rev., **16**:101–10, 1952.
101. Blair, E. B. Texas Rep. Biol. & Med., **8**:361, 1950.
102. Williams, O. B., and Reed, J. M. J. Infect. Dis., **71**:225–27, 1942.
103. Ohye, D. F., and Scott, W. J. Australian J. Biol. Sc., **6**:178–89, 1953.
104. Dolman, C. E., Chang, Helen, Kerr, Donna A., and Shearer, A. R. Canad. J. Pub. Health, **41**:215–29, 1950.
105. Olsen, A. M., and Scott, W. J. Australian J. Scient. Res., ser. B, **3**:219–33, 1950.
106. Sugiyama, H. J. Bact., **62**:81–96, 1951.
107. ———. Bact. Rev., **16**:125–26, 1952.
108. Dickson, E. C., Burke, G. S., Beck, D., Johnson, J., and King, H. J.A.M.A., **79**:1239–40, 1922.
109. Dickson, E. C. Proc. Soc. Exper. Biol. & Med., **25**:426–27, 1928.

110. MEYER, K. F. J. Prevent. Med., **5**:261–93, 1931.
111. FAUST, HILDA. Nutrition program during war: home canning. Agricultural Extension Service, U.S. Dept. Agr. and Univ. California, 1942.
112. TANNER, F. W., and OGLESBY, E. W. Food Res., **1**:481–94, 1936.
113. TANNER, F. W., BEAMER, P. R., and RICKHER, C. J. Food Res., **5**: 323–33, 1940.
114. COLLIER, R. E., and WYNNE, E. S. Unpublished data.
115. ANDERSEN, A. A. J. Bact., **64**:145–49, 1952.
116. CAMERON, E. J., and BOHRER, C. W. Food Technol., **8**:340–42, 1951.
117. WILLIAMS, O. B., and FLEMING, T. C. Antibiotics & Chemother., **2**: 75–78, 1952.
118. FOSTER, JACKSON W., and WYNNE, E. STATEN. J. Bact., **55**:495–501, 1948.
119. ROTH, NORMAN G., and HALVORSON, H. O. J. Bact., **63**:429–35, 1952.
120. WYNNE, E. STATEN, and FOSTER, JACKSON W. J. Bact., **55**:61–68, 1948.
121. ———. *Ibid.*, pp. 69–73.
122. SCOTT, W. J., and STEWART, D. F. J. Council Scient. & Indust. Res., **17**:16–22, 1944.
123. ———. *Ibid.*, **18**:173–80, 1945.
124. J. Dept. Agr., Union of South Africa, 1920; and eleventh and twelfth reports of the director of veterinary education and research, Part II, p. 1201. Dept. Agr., Union of South Africa, 1927.
125. South African J. M. Sc., **23**:520, 1926.
126. Rev. gin. de med. vit., **35**:193, 1927; and thirteenth and fourteenth reports of the director of veterinary research and education, Part I, p. 45. Dept. Agr., Union of South Africa, 1928.
127. NAKAMURA, Y., *et al.* Spec. Rep. Pub. Health Lab., Hokkaido, Japan, 1954.
128. SAITO, S., *et al.* J. Akita M. Sc., **6**:1, 1954.
129. PRÉVOT, A. R., and HUET, M. Bull. Acad. nat. méd., **25** and **26**:432, 1951.
130. HAZEN, ELIZABETH L. Proc. Soc. Exper. Biol. & Med., **50**:112–14, 1942.
131. WAGENAAR, R. O. Unpublished data, Food Research Institute.
132. BENGTSON, I. A. Pub. Health Rep., **37**:164–70, 1922.
133. KALMBACH, E. R. Science, **72**:658–60, 1930.
134. GILTNER, L. T., and COUCH, J. F. Science, **72**:660, 1930.
135. SHAW, R. M., and SIMPSON, GRETTA S. J. Bact., **32**:79–88, 1936.
136. GUNNISON, J. B., and MEYER, K. F. Proc. Soc. Exper. Biol. & Med., **26**:89, 1928.
137. COLEMAN, GEORGE E., and MEYER, K. F. J. Infect. Dis., **31**:622–49, 1922.
138. STARIN, WILLIAM A., and DACK, GAIL M. J. Infect. Dis., **36**:383–412, 1925.
139. LAMANNA, CARL, and LEWIS, CHARLES. J. Bact., **51**:398–99, 1946.
140. LEWIS, KEITH H., and HILL, EDWIN V. J. Bact., **53**:213–30, 1947.
141. ABRAMS, A., KEGELES, G., and HOTTLE, G. A. J. Biol. Chem., **164**: 63–79, 1946.

142. LAMANNA, C., McELROY, O. E., and EKLUND, H. W. Science, **103:** 613–14, 1946.
143. LAMANNA, CARL, EKLUND, HENNING W., and McELROY, OLIVE E. J. Bact., **52:**1–13, 1946.
144. KEGELES, G. J. Am. Chem. Soc., **68:**1670, 1946.
145. PUTNAM, F. W., LAMANNA, C., and SHARP, D. G. J. Biol. Chem., **165:**735–36, 1946.
146. WAGMAN, JACK, and BATEMAN, J. B. Arch. Biochem., **31:**424–30, 1951.
147. ———. *Ibid.*, **45:**375–83, 1953.
148. WAGMAN, JACK. Arch. Biochem., **50:**104–12, 1954.
149. BUEHLER, H. J., SCHANTZ, E. J., and LAMANNA, C. J. Biol. Chem., **169:**295–302, 1947.
150. LAMANNA, CARL. Proc. Soc. Exper. Biol. & Med., **69:**332–36, 1948.
151. LAMANNA, CARL, and LOWENTHAL, JOSEPH P. J. Bact., **61:**751–52, 1951.
152. LAMANNA, CARL, and GLASSMAN, HAROLD N. J. Bact., **54:**575–84, 1947.
153. NIGG, C., HOTTLE, G. A., CORIELL, L. L., ROSENWALD, A. S., and BEVERIDGE, G. W. J. Immunol., **55:**245–54, 1947.
154. HOTTLE, G. A., NIGG, C., and LICHTY, J. A. J. Immunol., **55:**255–62, 1947.
155. HOTTLE, G. A., and ABRAMS, A. J. Immunol., **55:**183–87, 1947.
156. REAMES, H. R., KADULL, P. J., HOUSEWRIGHT, R. D., and WILSON, J. B. J. Immunol., **55:**309–24, 1947.
157. LAMANNA, C., and JENSEN, W. I. Proc. Soc. Am. Bact., p. 106, 1952.
158. STERNE, M. Science, **119:**440–41, 1954.
159. WENTZEL, L. M., STERNE, M., and POLSON, A. NATURE, **166:**739, 1950.
160. THERBER, A., VILJOEN, P. R., GREEN, H. H., MEIER, H., and ROBINSON, E. M. Eleventh and twelfth reports of the director of veterinary education and research, Dept. Agr., Union of South Africa, Part II, pp. 1099–1201, 1927.
161. BENNETTS, H. W., and HALL, H. T. B. Australian Vet. J., **14:**105–18, 1938.
162. STERNE, M., and WENTZEL, L. M. J. Immunol., **65:**175–83, 1950.
163. BOROFF, DANIEL A., and CABEEN, HELEN DALE. J. Bact., **67:**198–201, 1954.
164. SCOTT, W. J., and STEWART, D. F. Australian J. Appl. Sc., **1:**188–99, 1950.
165. SCOTT, W. J. Australian J. Appl. Sc., **1:**200–207, 1950.

V *Staphylococcus Food Poisoning*

Staphylococcus food poisoning, like botulism, is produced by a toxin formed in the food before ingestion. It is probably the commonest of all food poisoning, although we have no knowledge of the number of cases occurring annually because it is not reportable. Staphylococcus food-poisoning symptoms are different from those of botulism; they appear more rapidly and are of shorter duration. Recovery is complete in the majority of cases. A physician may not always be summoned, and the next day the individual may be able to carry on his routine duties. Most afflicted persons are satisfied with the diagnosis of food poisoning or the incorrect diagnosis of "ptomaine poisoning." Inasmuch as this type of ailment involves many people at one time or another, not much attention is paid to staphylococcus food poisoning, and consequently it may soon be forgotten. When large groups of people are attacked at banquets, encampments, or public institutions, however, publicity is given, and action is taken to determine the cause of the illnesses.

Staphylococci are common organisms found in the throats of individuals, on their skin as a causative agent of pimples, boils, and carbuncles, and in great abundance in the postnasal drip of patients recovering from colds.

HISTORY

The question of how long staphylococcus food poisoning has afflicted man is conjectural. Although staphylococci were not recognized before 1880, when Pasteur (1) found them in pus, and they were not properly classified until 1884 (2), these organisms have undoubtedly caused food poisoning for centuries. A few examples of outbreaks taken from the literature will illustrate this point. In 1830 (3) the comment was made:

. . . certain articles of food have been frequently observed on the Continent to acquire poisonous qualities of a peculiar kind, and in a way which chemists and physicians have not hitherto been able to explain satisfactorily. Among these articles the most frequent are a peculiar variety of

109

sausage, and a particular kind of cheese used in Germany; but both in France and Germany bacon and ham have been also several times found to acquire poisonous qualities analogous to those which characterize the sausage-poison and cheese-poison. A very elaborate inquiry into an accident supposed to have arisen from spoiled ham has just been published by M. Ollivier in the Archives Générales de Médecine. His investigations set completely at rest the common notion that such accidents arise from the accidental impregnation of the meat with metallic poisons; but he has not succeeded in discovering the real cause.

In the instance which gave rise to his investigation, the master of a family purchased a ham pye at a pastry-cook's in Paris; and the whole family ate the meat of the pye the same day, and the crust on the following day. Three hours after dinner the master of the house was seized with general uneasiness, followed by cold sweats, shivering, violent pain in the stomach, and frequent vomiting; then with burning thirst, extreme tenderness of the belly, so that the weight of the bed-clothes could scarcely be borne, profuse purging, and colic of extreme violence. His daughter, twenty-seven years of age, and a child nine years old were similarly attacked. A physician who was called to their assistance soon after they were taken ill, drew up a minute report of the symptoms in each of his patients, and declared that they had a violent inflammation of the stomach, which he was inclined to ascribe to natural verdigris, or the carbonate of copper having been communicated by the pastry-cook's moulds. In a few days all the three individuals recovered under an antiphlogistic treatment. About the same period several accidents of the like nature occurred among the customers of this pastry-cook; and in consequence a judicial investigation was ordered. The shop being properly inspected it was found that every operation was conducted with due attention to cleanliness.

Chemical tests made of the meat and the paste separately and of the vomitus and stools did not reveal a trace of the commonly recognized chemical poisons—arsenic, copper, antimony, or lead.

In 1862 a food-poisoning outbreak caused by rabbit pie was described by John Buckenham (4) as follows:

On the 19th of August, a family of ten persons residing in this neighbourhood, having at dinner partaken of a rabbit-pie, were all shortly afterwards seized with diarrhoea and violent pains in the abdomen, which continued throughout the greater part of the night. Some astringent medicine having been administered, considerable relief was obtained. On the following morning, however, the precise cause of their illness not being suspected, several members of the family again partook of the remnant of the pie, reproducing the symptoms of the previous day in an alarmingly aggravated form, vomiting and violent cramps in the lower extremities being superadded.

Having been hastily summoned, I found on my arrival one of the patients in a state of collapse, pulseless, and insensible, and bathed in a cold, clammy perspiration. The others were also suffering more or less severely in proportion to the quantity of the poisonous food each person had eaten. . . .

From inquiries instituted in the matter, it has been ascertained beyond doubt that these sudden and remarkable symptoms were attributable solely to the rabbit-pie, as each person who partook of it was similarly affected, and the symptoms recurred in every instance in those who again ate of it, whilst those who partook more sparingly or avoided it escaped. The rabbits, and other materials composing the pie, it was proved were perfectly fresh and good, but were probably rendered unwholesome, though not unpalatable, by the process of cooking, having been baked beneath an impervious crust, which prevented the evaporation of the generated steam. It was afterwards permitted to stand for two or three days during very hot weather, which caused it to undergo a state of fermentation, as was observed from its peculiar appearance in the entire absence of jelly. Had the food been consumed when hot and freshly baked, or the confined steam freely permitted to escape by raising the paste, or otherwise affording sufficient ventilation, it is probable that no injurious effects would have resulted; at least such appears to me the only satisfactory explanation to account for the above remarkable symptoms.

An outbreak of food poisoning caused by eating pork brawn (molded product containing pieces of pork in a gelatin matrix made by prolonged cooking) was reported by Edward Mackey (5) in 1873:

Cases similar to the following deserve record, because they have a medico-legal interest, and may be required for reference and precedent.

On January 4th last, at Hampton-in-Arden, sixteen persons, including men, women, and children, aged from five to seventy-eight years, were suddenly attacked with violent vomiting and purging, accompanied in most cases with general and severe muscular cramps, soreness of eyes, and sense of burning and constriction in the throat. . . . Some seemed to be in serious danger; but, under appropriate treatment, all were convalescent next day. It was found that all had eaten some "pork brawn," and had begun to suffer two or three hours afterwards. All who had eaten any suffered more or less. The brawn had been bought from one provision-dealer in the village, a respectable man who could give no reason for its bad effects. He had eaten a little of it (perhaps two ounces), and had thought it particularly good. Of eighteen pounds made, six had been sold; the rest he himself gave into the custody of the police.

No mineral poisons were found in samples of the brawn subjected to chemical examination. In concluding, the author states:

I certified to the absence of mineral poison and to the probability of formation of acrid fatty acids—a suggestion previously made by Dr. Wade.

It may be observed in conclusion, that the dealer will never attempt brawn-making again, "for he suffered so much in his mind." His customers were considerate towards him, and no legal proceedings arose. Somewhat similar cases might not always end with as little mischief.

In 1879 Henry Leffmann (6), lecturer in toxicology in the summer school of Jefferson Medical College, called attention to the frequency with which cream puffs had been implicated in outbreaks of food poisoning. He wrote: "I have made chemical examinations of portions of cream puffs that have caused trouble, but have not found anything that could be assigned as the cause of the action."

Since 1880 numerous bacteria have been found to cause disease, and, as will be pointed out, the incrimination of staphylococci in food poisoning dates from that time.

Professor Victor C. Vaughan (7) in 1884 made the following statement with reference to food poisoning caused by cheese:

> It is well known that cases of severe illness follow the eating of some cheese. Indeed, such instances have been observed in various parts of the world for the past three hundred years. They are of frequent occurrence in the North German countries and in the United States. In England they are less frequently observed, while in France, where much cheese is used, we find no record of any such cases. In northern Ohio, a few years ago, the reputation of a large cheese factory is said to have been destroyed by the great number of cases of alarming illness occurring among those who ate of its product. In Michigan, during the past six months, nearly three hundred cases of cheese-poisoning have been reported.

Dr. Vaughan observed that the old, foul-smelling cheeses, such as Limburger and Schweitzer, are alkaline in reaction and that poisoning never results from their use.

Professor Vaughan performed the following experiments with samples of poisonous cheese:

> I covered some bits of the cheese with 90 per cent. alcohol, agitated thoroughly, and filtered. The clear alcoholic filtrate, on being evaporated at a low temperature, left a large residue of fatty acids with possibly some contained nitrogenous bases. Having ascertained that nothing could be learned by feeding the cheese to the lower animals, I determined to experiment upon myself. I ate a piece of this alcoholic extract, about the size of a hazelnut. It had a bitter, acrid taste, and in ten or fifteen minutes there were marked constriction and dryness of the fauces, much the same as that experienced while under the effect of atropia. Later there was considerable nausea, and I could readily believe that a larger amount would have caused vomiting. This experiment was repeated a number of times with the same result, and from it I conclude that the poisonous material, whatever it may be, is contained in the alcoholic extract. This would indicate a chemical poison and not a bacteric one. However, this chemical poison might be generated by the agency of bacteria. . . .
> Microscopical examination of the opalescent drops already mentioned,

or of water which had been poured upon the cheese and allowed to stand for a short time, revealed bacterium termo and spherical bodies from ¾ to 1 micromillimeter in diameter, the latter having a rapid swinging motion. These spherical bodies are not the ova of small animals, for they are insoluble in ammonium hydrate. They may be micrococci, or the resting spores, of some bacillus.

Henry B. Baker, secretary of the Michigan State Board of Health, in 1884 sent some of the cheese which had caused illness to Dr. George M. Sternberg (8), surgeon, United States Army, who was stationed at Johns Hopkins University. Dr. Sternberg found that fluid from the cavities of the cut cheese, on direct examination, showed the presence of micrococci and no bacilli or other microorganisms. Cultures in broth, when incubated at 38° C. for 24 hours, contained only micrococci in pairs and in chains.

Two rabbits inoculated subcutaneously with about 2 ml. of broth culture remained in good health. Rats and dogs fed the cheese developed no ill effects. A dog given 3 ml. of broth culture of the micrococcus and, subsequently, 10 ml. of an alcoholic extract of cheese remained well. However, Dr. Duggan, who assisted Dr. Sternberg with his experimental work, ate about 15 gm. of the cheese at 2:30 P.M., and at 5:00 P.M. he was attacked with nausea and vomiting and had one loose discharge from the bowels. He was not subject to similar attacks and ascribes the symptoms to the cheese which he had eaten. Dr. Sternberg concludes: "It seems not improbable that the poisonous principle is a ptomaine developed in the cheese as a result of the vital activity of the above mentioned micrococcus, or of some other microorganisms which had preceded it, and had perhaps been killed by its own poisonous products."

It is of interest that Dr. Sternberg in his book entitled *A Textbook of Bacteriology* (9), chapter v, "Ptomaines and Toxalbumins," discusses the problem of cheese poisoning under a paragraph headed "Tyrotoxicon" and states:

First obtained by Vaughan in poisonous cheese, and subsequently by the same chemist and others in poisonous milk and ice cream. Chemically tyrotoxicon is very unstable. It is decomposed when heated with water to 90° C. It is insoluble in ether. From sixteen kilogrammes of poisonous cheese Vaughan obtained 0.5 gramme of the poison. The symptoms produced in man by eating cheese or milk containing tyrotoxicon are vertigo, nausea, vomiting, and severe rigors, with pain in the bowels attended with purging, numbness and a pricking sensation in the limbs, and great prostration.

In the years following the reports by Vaughan and Sternberg, micrococci were found repeatedly in large numbers in foods involved in food-poisoning outbreaks. Thus Denys (10) in 1894 found them in beef; Owen (11) in 1906 recovered them in dried beef; and Barber's (12) classic work incriminated them in milk.

A commission (10) reported the work of Dr. Denys, who was a professor at the University of Louvain. According to Dr. Denys, all except one child in a family ate meat from a cow dead of "vitullary fever," and, while the child remained well, the others became sick, and one death resulted from an illness resembling cholera. Bacteriological examination led him to conclude that the trouble was due to the presence of pyogenic staphylococci. Furthermore, he ascertained that cultures of the organism exerted little or no effect when injected into the pleura of rabbits, and the commission itself ventured to state that the route of administration may be important. Owen (11) corroborated the findings of Denys by reporting the acute intestinal intoxication within a few days of nineteen people in Kalamazoo, Michigan. The symptoms, characteristic of staphylococcus food poisoning, were enumerated in detail, and the board of health incriminated dried beef, which appeared from subsequent work to have become contaminated after it reached the particular store in which it was sold. The meat was normal in odor and in appearance, except for a slight greenish tinge in a few places. Detailed work by Dr. Novy indicated that cultures from this meat produced little or no effect when fed to various laboratory animals.

This subject was reopened in 1914 by Barber (12). Suffice it to say that he found that milk drawn from one-quarter of the udder of a cow which had been the seat of an attack of mastitis 3 years previously contained a white staphylococcus which was responsible for sporadic cases of acute gastrointestinal upsets on a certain farm in the Philippine Islands during the years 1909–13. This organism developed in sufficient numbers to be serious only in unrefrigerated milk or cream. It was small, tended to form diplococci, and liberated a toxic substance which was responsible for the upsets. No agglutinins were formed in the serum of those affected, and, as previously, animals, including monkeys, exhibited no symptoms upon ingesting large quantities of milk cultures. The findings in this excellent report remained unappreciated for 15 years. The significance of this work incriminating staphylococci was not recognized, and food poisoning was, with few exceptions, ascribed to other bacterial agents. For example, in World War I, 2,000 soldiers in the German army suffered an illness characterized by vomiting, diarrhea, and exhaustion, with symptoms appearing within 2–3 hours after eating sausage (13). The sausage was subsequently shown to contain cocci in large numbers and *Proteus vulgaris*. The investigator assigned the causative role to *P. vulgaris*.

In 1929 the role of staphylococci in food poisoning was rediscovered when Dr. W. E. Cary (14) brought to the laboratory two Christmas cakes which had been submitted to him by two of his physician-friends who knew he was interested in food poisoning. These three-layer sponge cakes had a thick cream filling and had been ornately iced and decorated with chopped pistachio nuts and maraschino cherries. They had been baked on December 23 or 24 in a commercial Italian bakery in Chicago and were delivered on the afternoon of the twenty-fourth. The cakes were presumably refrigerated at the bakery but were not kept in iceboxes later. One cake had been served at various times on the twenty-sixth to 5 adults and 3 children and the other at dinner to 3 adults. The 11 individuals who ate the cakes became ill. The victims were from four families, so that other items of food could easily be eliminated. More than half of each cake was available for laboratory study, and work was begun 15 hours after the cakes were first cut.

Four monkeys were fed a saline suspension of the entire cake by stomach tube, and 3 mice received a saline suspension of the cake substance orally. None showed ill effects. Since the heavy metals, mercury and arsenic, were not found in the cake and no *Salmonella* organisms were isolated when appropriate cultures were made, the logical alternative left was to test the material on human volunteers. It was thereafter found that the sponge cake, after removal of the frosting and filler, was responsible for the trouble.

A bacteriological examination of the cake substance revealed 19 different types of colonies. The predominant 3 were further studied. A filtrate from a veal-infusion broth culture of only one of these, incubated for 40 hours, caused a rabbit, when injected intravenously with 4 ml. of the filtrate, to develop a profuse watery diarrhea, to lose 170 gm. of its body weight (7 per cent) in 5 hours, and to die

12 hours later. In addition, 3 human volunteers drank, respectively, 25, 10, and 5 ml. of the filtrate which was lethal to the rabbit. Typical symptoms, beginning after 3 hours, occurred in the volunteer drinking the 25-ml. portion. The volunteers who took the smaller amounts of filtrate (10 and 5 ml.) experienced minor sensations of nausea, chilliness, and gastrointestinal distress after 3 hours. The organism from which the toxic filtrate was prepared was a yellow hemolytic staphylococcus and, in smears from broth cultures, was arranged in pairs or chains rather than in clusters, like many of the staphylococci. In this respect, the morphology agreed with Barber's (12) description.

The proof of the causative role of staphylococci in food poisoning has rested upon experiments with human volunteers, since none of the ordinary laboratory animals are susceptible to feeding of enterotoxin in amounts which affect man. The long delay in recognition of the role of this organism in food poisoning may be attributed chiefly to the immense amount of publicity given *Salmonella* or paratyphoid organisms in food poisoning. In fact, when in earlier outbreaks *Salmonella* was not found, various methods (discussed under "*Salmonella*") were devised to detect their heat-stable products, for it was falsely assumed that they gave rise to food-poisoning symptoms in man. Paradoxically, perhaps, knowledge of the ubiquity of the staphylococcus has contributed to the delay in the recognition of its importance in food poisoning.

The "modern era" of staphylococcus food poisoning dates from 1930. Since that time our knowledge of the subject has increased rapidly, and this most common of all types of food poisoning is now recognized throughout the civilized world.

EPIDEMIOLOGY

The conditions necessary for an outbreak of staphylococcus food poisoning are as follows: contamination of a food with enterotoxin-producing staphylococci, a suitable food in which the organism can grow, and the keeping of this food for a sufficient time at a temperature compatible with growth.

Many different types of foods have been involved in staphylococcus food poisoning. Ham pie, rabbit pie, pork brawn, cream puffs, cheese, beef, dried beef, milk, sausage, and cream-filled cake have already been mentioned. Kelly and Dack (15) list outbreaks due to cream-filled éclairs and tarts, custard-filled doughnuts, chocolate éclairs, milk, chicken gravy, and tongue sandwiches. In addition, other foods have been incriminated, such as ham or tongue (16), hollandaise sauce (17), *kamaboko* (fish sausage) (18), liver sausage (19), goat's milk (20), pressed pickled beef (21), ice cream (22), chicken salad (23), pineapple trifle (24), and bread pudding (25). Outbreaks have been reported in newspapers where potato salad was the food implicated. Wethington and Fabian (26) state that mayonnaise and salad dressing are not probable sources of staphylococcus food poisoning because of their content of acetic acid. Although salad dressing used by itself may not be a medium for growth of staphylococci, it produces an excellent medium in potato salad.

Fuchs (27) studied outbreaks in 1939 from water, milk, and other foods. He found large numbers were reported by a few states and a smaller number or none from others. The reporting of these outbreaks was out of proportion to the relative population of the states. Fuchs notes:

> For example, 1 state, with only one-tenth of the country's population, reported practically one-half of all the water-borne outbreaks. Again, 3 states reported over one-half of all the milk-borne outbreaks. Similarly, two states accounted for more than half of all the food-borne outbreaks. From our knowledge of the quality and extent of the public health activities of these states it would be unreasonable to assume that they are below average in environmental sanitation. On the contrary, the logical explanation probably lies in their efficient epidemiological organization for uncovering outbreaks and in their willingness to report such outbreaks [27].

For the year 1939 outbreaks of food poisoning traced to pies and pastries were the most numerous, with those due to pork and pork products second in occurrence. Fuchs does not state the number in this group due to staphylococci or to other causes. In upstate New York from 1935 to 1939, 17 outbreaks (1,246 cases) (28) of staphylococcus food poisoning reported were due to cream-filled bakery goods. In one of these outbreaks 700 individuals were involved.

Feig (29), in a study of outbreaks of food poisoning reported to the United States Public Health Service for the years from 1945 to 1947, observed that 82.2 per cent, in which the etiological agent was determined, were due to staphylococci. In 1951, 63 outbreaks of food poisoning (30) in which the presence of staphylococci was demonstrated were reported to the Public Health Service. In 1952, 77 outbreaks with 3,798 cases were reported (31), and, in 1953, 81 outbreaks with 4,045 cases were reported. The slight increase in outbreaks (32) from year to year may be due to physicians' becoming more aware of this type of food poisoning. Obviously, only the more dramatic episodes in which outbreaks occur among large gatherings of people are reported, but these are of small statistical value in determining the frequency of staphylococcus food-poisoning outbreaks in small groups or in the home.

In England most outbreaks of food poisoning reported have been alleged to be due to *Salmonella*. However, Wilson (33) states:

> There is no exact information on the frequency of food poisoning in this country. The disease is not notifiable, cases are often sporadic, the true nature may not be recognized, and the illness may be so transient that no doctor is called in. Available evidence suggests that the disease is common, but that the great majority of sporadic cases and many of the smaller outbreaks never come to the notice of the health authorities. Before the war, Scott estimated that about one-third of all cases of food poisoning were of the staphylococcal toxin type.

In England and Wales for the years 1941 through 1948 a total of 90 outbreaks, varying in number from 6 to 20 per cent (34), of staphylococcus food poisoning were reported; in 1949, 97 outbreaks (35); in 1950 (36), 82; in 1951, 65; and in 1952, 82 (37). The sharp rise in 1949 and later years may have been due again to better recognition and reporting of this type of food poisoning rather than to a change in the incidence of the outbreaks. From 1949 through 1952 staphylococcus food-poisoning outbreaks in England and Wales accounted for approximately 2 per cent of all reported.

In other countries of the world staphylococcus food-poisoning outbreaks are being detailed in the literature with increasing frequency, but no information is available as to the true incidence. Fish sausage (18) is referred to by the Japanese. Timmerman (19) in Holland describes an outbreak due to liver sausage. He tested a filtrate, from the staphylococcus involved, on a human volunteer, who developed symptoms of acute food poisoning. He is of the opinion that a larger number of cases of food poisoning are caused by staphylococci than is generally believed and that poisonings that develop after the eating of cheese are often caused by these organisms. Timmerman discounts the role of *Escherichia coli* in cheese poisoning, because *E. coli* is present in almost 60 per cent of samples of cheese and causes no poisoning.

The growth requirements of the staphylococci are easily fulfilled in many different types of food. Custard-filled bakery goods are probably responsible for the greatest number of outbreaks, while ham and tongue rank next. Slocum and Linden (16) found that the consumption of "ready-to-eat" hams or tongue was responsible for 20 outbreaks of food poisoning, apparently due to staphylococci, in which at least 1,028 individuals were affected. Tipton and Smiley (38) reported 3,884 cases in 6 outbreaks occurring in the Navy which were traced to ham.

Hauge (39) has reviewed the literature on the significance of staphylococci in milk. In his examination of 124 samples from several farms supplying milk to Oslo, Norway, he found 45 per cent to contain yellow hemolytic staphylococci, with 60.6 per cent of the strains coagulase-positive. Staphylococci are a common cause of mastitis in cattle and, next to *Streptococcus agalactiae*, are considered by Plastridge *et al.* (40) and Little and Plastridge (41) to be the most frequent cause of chronic mastitis in cattle. Slanetz and Bartley (42) have found herds of dairy cows in which staphylococci produced a greater incidence of infection than did *S. agalactiae*. In an experimental herd they found that approximately 20 per cent of the uninfected quarters of cows' udders became infected with mastitis staphylococci each year during a 5-year period.

Bacteriophages for strains of *Staphylococcus aureus* were studied by Burnet and Lush (43) with the idea of grouping or classifying the strains. Fisk (44) developed methods for isolating and cultivating phages from *S. aureus*. Blair and Carr (45) have reviewed the literature and presented an excellent discussion on the methodology of the bacteriophage typing of staphylococci. In England a staphylococcal reference laboratory has been established at the Central Public Health Laboratory at Colindale. With some 21 type strains of staphylococcal bacteriophages, strains of staphylococci isolated from incriminated foods in food-poisoning outbreaks have been typed and compared with strains from food handlers. By this method the source of contamination has been tentatively identified (22, 46, 47). Re-

peated outbreaks have sometimes been traced to the same food
handler (22).

SYMPTOMS

The symptoms of staphylococcus food poisoning appear in about
3 hours, occasionally in from 1 to 6 hours, after ingesting food containing the enterotoxin. The incubation period is influenced by the
amount of enterotoxin consumed and the susceptibility of the individual. Usually, the first symptom observed is salivation, which is
subsequently followed by nausea, vomiting, retching, abdominal
cramping of varying severity, and diarrhea. In severe cases blood
and mucus may be observed in the stools and vomitus. In mild cases
there may be nausea and vomiting without diarrhea, or there may
be cramping and diarrhea without vomiting. Headache, muscular
cramping, and sweating often occur if symptoms are moderately
severe. Marked prostration accompanies the vomiting and diarrhea
in severe cases. In such cases fever may occur, or the temperature
may be subnormal. Denison (48) reported one case in which the
temperature dropped from 98°6 to 96°0 F. and returned to normal
after 9 hours. The blood pressure in this same case dropped from
120/80 to 60/40. Although staphylococcus food poisoning in otherwise normal individuals is usually not fatal, a few fatalities have
occurred where inadequate treatment was given. For example,
Denys (10) reports the death of one member of a family made ill
from contaminated beef, the illness resembling cholera. In another
outbreak 2 children, three and four years old, died within 24 hours
after each drank 250 cc. of milk from a goat suffering from acute
suppurative mastitis due to *S. aureus* (20). In normal cases recovery
is usually rapid in from 1 to 3 days. Some patients, however, may
not completely recover for a week or more. Individuals may vary
considerably in their susceptibility to the enterotoxin. One human
volunteer (49) vomited after the ingestion of 0.5 ml. of the filtrate
of a staphylococcus culture and was nauseated on one occasion by
only 0.25 ml. This filtrate was fed in increasing doses up to 13 ml.
to another volunteer without causing active symptoms. In another
experiment (15) involving a sandwich contaminated with staphylococci, one individual became severely ill, although another was not
affected. Therefore, since susceptibility among different individuals

varies, the size of the dose of the enterotoxin is not the only factor
determining the severity of symptoms. Similar data from reported
attacks have been assembled in Table 9. The data are fairly reliable,
since, for the most part, single families were involved and the incriminated food was uniform.

Because some individuals do not develop symptoms of food
poisoning when they ingest staphylococcus enterotoxin, the question
arises as to the relative susceptibility of the population. There are,

TABLE 9

SUSCEPTIBILITY OF INDIVIDUALS TO STAPHYLO-
COCCUS FOOD POISONING

Outbreak	No. of People Eating In- criminated Food	No. Ill	Per Cent Ill
1. (48)	11	11	100
2. (50)	325	....	60–70
3. (51)	3	3	100
4. (52) Family P	4	4	100
Family W	3	3	100
Family B	4	4	100
Family B (No. 2)	4	3	75
Family O	6	6	100
5. (53) Family M	2	2	100
L luncheon	5 or 6	5	82–100
Family T	2	2	100
Family P	4	4	100
Family McQ	5	5	100
6. (54)	102	96	94.1

unfortunately, many sources of error in obtaining information
when large numbers of people are involved. The food implicated
may not contain enterotoxin at the time of distribution but may
develop it later under suitable conditions of time and temperature.
It may be kept by one housewife for a period of time and at a temperature different from that of another homemaker. Accordingly, a
single outbreak involving the same item of food from a central
source will not contain a standard amount of enterotoxin with which
to judge the relative susceptibility of individuals in a large outbreak.
Another source of error is the difficulty in obtaining accurate data
from a large number of people. It is sometimes impossible for
one investigator to see all the persons involved. Also, the amounts of

items of food eaten vary with the individual, so that the dosage may not be uniform even in a family group. Finally, outbreaks in which only one or two in a family are affected are probably never reported. From the data it is evident, however, that when entero-toxin is ingested in food, few people escape illness.

TREATMENT

In staphylococcus food poisoning, vomiting and diarrhea are generally severe, and it is unnecessary to empty the stomach with a stomach pump or give cathartics to free the rest of the gastrointesti-nal tract of enterotoxin. In severe cases prostration is acute, and blood pressures of 60/20 have been observed. In fatal cases, circula-tory collapse occurs. The symptoms of shock are due in part to the loss of body fluids, resulting in dehydration and disturbances of salt balance and should be counterbalanced by giving normal saline solu-tions parenterally. The amount of fluid given should be governed by the age of the patient and the severity of the vomiting and diarrhea. No specific drug or serum therapy is of value.

LABORATORY DIAGNOSIS OF OUTBREAKS OF STAPHYLOCOCCUS
   FOOD POISONING

One of the most characteristic features of staphylococcus food poisoning is the shortness of the time interval between eating the incriminated food and the onset of symptoms. This incubation period may vary from 1 to 6 hours but is generally about $2\frac{1}{2}$–3 hours. If an outbreak of food poisoning occurs within this incubation period, it is helpful to the laboratory worker to have the epidemiological evi-dence regarding the suspected items of food. By submitting a list of foods served at the meal in question, together with the number of individuals ill and the number not ill, specific items of food involved can often be determined. Much time can thereby be saved in search-ing for the causative agent in the specific food or foods common to those who were sick.

Weighed samples of solid food and measured samples of liquid food are used to ascertain the types of bacteria present. The solid food is ground in a sterile mortar with sterile sand and saline. Deci-mal dilutions of the food samples are made and plated in veal-infusion agar. The plates are counted at the end of 24 and 48 hours.

Blood agar plates and selective media (eosin–methylene blue or *Salmonella-Shigella* agar) are streaked to rule out gram-negative intestinal pathogenic organisms, such as *Shigella* and *Salmonella* types.

In the case of staphylococcus food poisoning the involved food usually contains hundreds of millions of staphylococci per gram. Staphylococcus food poisoning may occur from food in which the organisms, after growing and producing enterotoxin, are destroyed by heating prior to serving. An example is an outbreak (55) in which all people using boiled milk in coffee became ill. Staphylococci were found in large numbers in the unboiled milk, leaving the enterotoxin. Another outbreak is reported which involved cooked as well as uncooked food. In this outbreak, of 160 persons (18) who ate *kamaboko* (fish sausage), 110 were poisoned, including 16 who thoroughly heated the sausage. The time and temperature of heating were not given, but apparently the food was sufficiently heated to destroy the staphylococci but not the enterotoxin. If the majority of people eating the food are affected, if hundreds of millions of staphylococci are present, and if the incubation period from the time of eating to the development of symptoms is $2\frac{1}{2}$–3 hours, the outbreak is almost certainly due to staphylococcus food poisoning. Circumstantial evidence, however, is not usually as precise. For example, an amount of enterotoxin may be formed so minute that it will be sufficient to affect only the most susceptible individuals. Staphylococci are ubiquitous, and millions are contained in many of our foods without causing illness, because many strains do not produce enterotoxin. On the other hand, food-poisoning strains do not produce potent enterotoxin in some foods.

The ideal and conclusive test for identifying staphylococcus food poisoning would be to detect enterotoxin in the food directly, but this has not as yet been developed by chemical or other laboratory methods. Small amounts of toxin may be detected only by using the highly susceptible human volunteer. The next best step, if large numbers of staphylococci are found, is to determine whether they are able to produce enterotoxin under experimental conditions.

Evans (56), Evans and Niven (57), and Evans, Buettner, and Niven (58) have studied a large number of strains of staphylococci, and they found that, without exception, the enterotoxigenic strains comprised an extremely homogeneous group. All enterotoxigenic strains produce coagulase, but not all coagulase-positive strains produce enterotoxin. On the other hand, without exception, all coagulase-negative cultures of staphylococci which Evans *et al.* have studied have failed to produce enterotoxin. On the basis of these studies, if a strain is coagulase-negative it may be considered non-enterotoxigenic. Therefore, the coagulase test should be a necessary part of the laboratory procedure in studying cultures from foods implicated in outbreaks of food poisoning.

Staphylococci are grown in Kolle flasks containing 75 ml. of 1 per cent veal-infusion agar of pH 6.0 (59). The flasks are placed in vacuum desiccator jars, the jars are partially exhausted, and 20 per cent carbon dioxide is admitted. After an incubation of 48–72 hours at 37° C., the agar is removed from the flask and squeezed through four layers of gauze. The fluid portion is then centrifuged at high speed to remove agar and most of the bacteria. It may then be filtered through a Berkefeld "N" or Seitz filter, or it may be fed directly to monkeys without filtration. A simplified medium for enterotoxin production has been prepared by Favorite and Hammon (60) (see accompanying table). The pH is adjusted to 7.6 with 40 per

	Amount per 100 Ml.
Casein hydrolysate	1.5 gm.
Thiamin chloride (vitamin B_1)	0.5 γ
Nicotinic acid	120.0 γ
Distilled water to a volume of	90.0 ml.
Phenol red (0.2 per cent)	0.4 ml.

cent sodium hydroxide, and the volume of the medium is brought to 99 ml. It is then autoclaved for 10 minutes at 10 pounds pressure. When cool, 1 ml. (0.25 gm.) of sterile 25 per cent glucose is added. The medium is poured into hexagonal, narrow-necked Pyrex nursing bottles of 250-ml. capacity. After inoculation, the bottles are placed in a large anaerobic jar from which all but 5 per cent of air has been removed and replaced by a carbon dioxide–oxygen mixture. As soon as the jar is opened, the cotton plugs of the bottles are quickly replaced with rubber stoppers. The bottles are slowly rotated during incubation. Enterotoxin is produced in this medium under these conditions in an amount equal to that produced in semisolid veal-infusion agar in an environment of 20 per cent carbon dioxide.

Surgalla *et al.* (61) employed three methods for producing large volumes of enterotoxin. The medium containing hydrolyzed casein was distributed in (1) Roux bottles, each containing 200 ml.; (2) 10 liters in 12-gallon bottles; and (3) bottles containing 1–15 liters. The Roux bottles were filled in batches of 50, seeded, and incubated at 37° C. in a sealed incubator containing 20 per cent carbon dioxide and 80 per cent air. The 10-liter quantities of medium in the 12-gallon bottles were seeded with culture and stoppered after the air was partially exhausted and replaced by 20 per cent carbon dioxide. The bottles were turned continuously on horizontal rollers during incubation at 37° C. Those containing 1–15 liters of medium were seeded and aerated with either air or a 20 per cent carbon dioxide plus 80 per cent oxygen gas mixture during incubation at 37° C.

The test for enterotoxin is made by feeding whole cultures or filtrates or by injecting boiled cultures or filtrates into the abdominal cavity or blood stream of animals. The amount of enterotoxin in such mixtures must be large if it is to be tested by this method, because no experimental animal has been found that will react to the small amounts of enterotoxin sufficient to cause severe reactions in man.

The rhesus monkey appears to be the best test animal to feed or inject with potent enterotoxin. Jordan and McBroom (62) found that *Macaca mulatta* reacts similarly to man when fed filtrates containing enterotoxin in amounts as small as 2–5 ml. and reacts more uniformly with larger doses. The usual procedure involves giving the monkey 50 ml. of culture or filtrate by stomach tube. Woolpert and Dack (59) made this statement:

Usually about an hour and a half after feeding, the animal becomes somewhat pale; increased salivation and swallowing movements are noted; the monkey may bend over in the corner of its cage with its forearms folded across its abdomen. The pallor and salivation increase; there is usually a short premonitory period marked by regurgitation. At about the beginning of the third hour vomiting sets in. This may be mild but is often profuse and projectile. Paroxysms of vomiting are apt to recur over a period of an hour or so. During this time the animal is very pallid and abject. Diarrhea may be a marked feature; in two cases in which large amounts of toxic material were fed, there was profuse diarrhea without vomiting; similar reactions have been noted in man. Recovery sets in rather abruptly after several hours, and on the following day the monkey may appear normal except for loss of weight. All of the animals that were fed recovered, although in a few instances diarrhea persisted several days.

Jordan and McBroom (62) also used the red spider (*Ateles geoffroyi*), *black spider* (*A. ater*), black howler (*Alouatta palliata inconsonans*), and white-throated monkeys (*Cebus capucinus capucinus*). These animals exhibited definite symptoms of diarrhea, lack of appetite, and malaise, and, in one instance, vomitus was found on the floor of the cage. Subsequently, Davison, Dack, and Cary (63) found that vomiting and other typical symptoms regularly follow the intravenous injection of rhesus monkeys with boiled filtrates from cultures of food-poisoning staphylococci in doses of 1 ml. per kilogram of body weight. Symptoms have also been produced with as small an amount as 0.2 ml. per kilogram.

Surgalla, Bergdoll, and Dack (64) reported results of feeding staphylococcus enterotoxin by stomach tube to approximately 1,000 *M. mulatta*. The relative susceptibility of the monkeys was predictable to some degree on the basis of past response to enterotoxin, but a wide variation was found. Unless new animals were used, graded dosage-response curves were unsatisfactory. Only on rare occasions was unprovoked emesis observed.

One disadvantage of using monkeys is that they are expensive to buy and to maintain. Another important objection is their resistance to the oral administration of enterotoxin as compared to the relative susceptibility of man. In addition, the monkey is not as easily handled as many other animals and is likely to become resistant to enterotoxin after several feedings. A source of error in these tests has been pointed out by Minett, who states: "Monkeys frequently regurgitate material into the mouth and then slowly swallow it, but it is doubtful if any significance should be attached to this act, since it was observed at times after unsown filtrate had been fed" (65). It may be that some of the discrepancies in the results reported by different investigators are explainable upon this basis.

The cat has also been extensively used in testing for staphylococcus enterotoxin. Dolman, Wilson, and Cockcroft (66) stated: "The cat is more akin to human beings than are rodents in dietary and excretory habits; is less prone to vomit than the dog; and is a more convenient and economical experimental animal than the monkey." These workers prepare filtrates by inoculating plates of semisolid nutrient agar medium with the strain of staphylococcus under investigation and harvesting them after 40 hours' incubation at 37° C. in an atmosphere of 30 per cent carbon dioxide and 70 per cent oxygen. The suspension is freed from agar by being passed through cheesecloth and filtered through a Seitz filter. To the filtrate, 0.3 per cent solution of formaldehyde (U.S.P.) is added, and the formalinized filtrate is kept in the incubator at 37° C. until rabbit and sheep cell hemolysins (alpha [α] and beta [β] toxins) are no longer detectable. The solution is then ready to test on kittens for the presence of enterotoxin. Davison *et al.* make this statement:

> In our more recent experiments, advantage has been taken of the greater heat stability of the enterotoxin as compared with the alpha and beta toxins. Filtrates have been placed in a boiling water bath for ½ hour prior to injection. Only negligible amounts of alpha and beta toxins survive this treatment, but enterotoxin, where present, proves heat-stable [63].

These workers observed that as little as 0.5 ml. of a potent filtrate injected intraperitoneally will cause a severe reaction in a 6–8-week-old kitten weighing 350–550 gm., while 3 ml. of a filtrate from innocuous strains or of formalinized broth will cause no upset, and also that adult cats may be used for the test but are harder to handle and appear relatively less sensitive than kittens.

Surgalla and Hite (67) made a comparative study of the production of enterotoxin and of alpha and beta hemolysins by a number of strains of staphylococci. They found that all the strains which were enterotoxic when fed to monkeys also produced alpha lysin, whereas only some of the cultures produced beta lysin. They concluded that staphylococcal enterotoxin and hemolysins are separable and distinct entities.

Kupchik (68) essentially substantiated this work, while others discovered that uninoculated medium alone produced symptoms in kittens (69). The fact that the intraperitoneal injection of sterile broth into kittens may give rise to food-poisoning symptoms is sufficient warning that each test should be controlled by injecting the test kitten with sterile broth first to see whether a reaction is elicited. If no food-poisoning symptoms follow, then unknown boiled cultures or filtrates prepared from the same medium may be tested. The reaction following the injection of kittens with sterile broth may or may not be due to peritoneal irritation. Certainly, our bacteriological media contain a complex mixture of chemicals. No two brands of peptone are alike, and no two lots of the same brand are identical chemically. The reactions occurring with sterile broth may well be due to the toxicity of the medium itself. Whether the simplified medium recommended by Favorite and Hammon (60) will prove practicable and obviate this difficulty is problematical.

Davison, Dack, and Cary (63) found that the assay of enterotoxic substances by the intravenous injection of kittens with specimens to be tested offers certain advantages. Since, as in monkeys, it is a more delicate test, only a small inoculum is required, and susceptible animals can be used repeatedly. Hammon is enthusiastic about this method and says:

> It would appear from the results of this study that the intravenous cat test for enterotoxin is one which can be readily applied to heat treated culture filtrates in any health department laboratory. Since adult cats or large kittens can be used, no difficulty should be encountered in acquiring and keeping the necessary animals, and each may be used three or four times before developing too great a tolerance. Negative results, however, should be confirmed by inoculation of at least two previously unused animals. A healthy cat, given a meal shortly before inoculation, should react by actually vomiting before any test is considered positive. This method of inoculation has definite advantages over the intra-abdominal route [70].

This test must, however, be used on a large scale in many laboratories before its true merits can be assessed. The introduction into the blood stream of various protein degradation products, as found in the ordinary laboratory media, may give rise to false positive tests similar to the intraperitoneal kitten experiments.

Robinton (71, 72) reported that decerebrated frogs (*Rana pipiens*) injected intraperitoneally with enterotoxin developed reverse peristalsis of the stomach. Reactions were found to occur with known emetic and enterotoxigenic substances and were reported to follow in 1–30 minutes after intragastric injection, depending upon the concentration of enterotoxin. Eddy (73), who was not able to confirm Robinton's work, concluded that the occurrence of a gastric spasm in frogs fed staphylococcal culture products is either a nonspecific response to various substances of an especially viscid nature, elicited more readily at certain seasons, or a response at one season to some undetermined stimulus. According to Surgalla, Bergdoll, and Dack (64), the frog test is unreliable for the detection of enterotoxin; the reverse peristaltic gastric waves were seen in frogs fed saline and other nonenterotoxic materials. When enterotoxin was fed, the reaction was unrelated to dosage.

Other animals used to test staphylococcus enterotoxin include white mice, wild mice, white rats, guinea pigs, rabbits, puppies, dogs, and canaries. Many of these species do not have a vomiting reflex, and diarrhea has been used as a criterion of reaction. At the November, 1941, meeting of the Society of Illinois Bacteriologists, Drs. Hopkins and Poland reported that young pigs are good test animals. They injected boiled staphylococcus filtrates intraperitoneally into young pigs and observed retching in a large majority. They also found that sensitivity to enterotoxin was retained after two or more injections.

CONTROL OF STAPHYLOCOCCUS FOOD POISONING

One of the important problems of the public health worker is the control of staphylococcus food poisoning. Staphylococci are abundant in nature, are carried in the throat, and are found in great numbers in the postnasal discharge following common colds. They cause pimples and carbuncles and other infections in man and may be isolated from the air of rooms. Fortunately, not all strains produce enterotoxin, and not all foods are favorable media. Nevertheless, it is obvious that foods exposed to the air may become contaminated with this coccus. Therefore, because some foods serve as excellent nutrient media for staphylococci, conditions should be made unfavorable for the production of enterotoxin. This may be accomplished simply by refrigeration; Segalove and Dack (74) have shown that enterotoxin is not formed in periods up to 4 weeks at a temperature of 4°–6°7 C., although other conditions necessary for enterotoxin production are fulfilled.

One of the more practical difficulties is the education of the public. If a food does not smell or taste spoiled, the layman thinks it safe for eating. The reverse is, unfortunately, often true. In the case of staphylococcus food poisoning, the product may contain sufficient enterotoxin to produce violent illness and yet have no odor of spoilage or abnormal taste. One group of foods which has given rise to numerous outbreaks of food poisoning is custard-filled bakery goods. Stritar, Dack, and Jungewaelter (75) worked out a simple method of reheating custard-filled puffs (pastry shells filled with custard) and éclairs (small oblong cakes filled with flavored custard and glazed over or frosted) for a period of time and at a temperature sufficient to kill staphylococci without impairing the flavor or appearance. At a temperature of 190.°6 C. (375° F.), for 30 minutes, the puff or éclair is not damaged, although exposed directly to this oven heat. The baker needs only to return filled shells to the oven in an ordinary pan. At higher temperatures excessive browning occurs unless egg whites are substituted for milk in the manufacture of the shell. A recommendation for routine use would be 30 minutes at temperatures ranging from 190.°6 C. (375° F.) to 218.°3 C. (425° F.). This principle of heating foods is old, and its public health significance has been well established, as, for example, in the pasteurization of milk. Korff (76) reported that about fifteen bakeries in Baltimore were reheating custard-filled pastries in 1936 and finding it satisfactory. Gilcreas and Coleman (77) recommended reheating custard filling in éclair shells for 15 minutes at a temperature of 216°–220° C. (420°–428° F.). They reported that rebaking éclairs, chocolate cream pie, and Boston cream pie for 20 minutes at 216° C. did not impair the appearance or palatability of the pastries. They concluded: "The adoption of this procedure in bakeries should reduce greatly the incidence of food poisoning induced by the enterotoxins of staphylococci in custard-filled products." Food poisoning from bakery goods is still prevalent. Unfortunately, many individuals do not change their long-established methods until they suffer personally.

Castellani (78), in a survey of bacteriostatic agents for staphylococci in cream pastry fillings, discovered that thioglycollic acid, DL-serine, L-cysteine, and glycine exerted bacteriostatic action on staphylococci in the descending order listed. Because of organoleptic and bacteriostatic considerations, DL-serine (0.2–0.3 per cent) appeared to offer the most promise. The inhibition is transient and is affected by the type of ingredients. If milk is omitted from the formula for custard, serine is more effective; if, instead, egg is omitted, it is even more effective. Shortening appears to have no effect, but coconut (79) completely overcomes the inhibitory effect of serine against staphylococci. The inhibitory effect of serine is pronounced after 24 hours' incubation at 86° F. but is slight after 48 hours. In custard filling its inhibitory effect is present on the indigenous flora as well as on staphylococci but is not effective against enterococci or *Salmonella* experimentally inoculated into custard filling.

Some bakeries have encountered more than one outbreak of staphylococcus food poisoning, and an attempt has been made in certain laboratories to look for carriers of food-poisoning staphylococci among bakery employees. Roberts and Wilson (80) conducted laboratory investigations over a period of a year on the personnel of one bakery. In an outbreak in March, 1938, they found that a strain of staphylococcus isolated from toxic pastry was the same as that in the nose and throat of the incriminated bakery owner. This man harbored the same strain from March, 1938, to April, 1939, despite medical treatment. According to Roberts and Wilson:

This person had apparently conveyed infection to other members of the bakery staff and to the utensils and food; and the same strain of staphylococcus was isolated from the cream-filled pastry on both occasions. It is of further interest to note that the persons implicated in each outbreak showed no visible signs of infection. This fact is rather disturbing when one considers the control of this type of food poisoning. Figures quoted by several authors show that the incidence of staphylococci in the noses of the general population is high. The proportion of these strains that may produce food poisoning is not known with certainty, but several surveys of strains from various sources indicate that roughly 40 per cent of these are enterotoxigenic, as shown by the kitten test. If these observations be true, the probability of food contamination, with possible food intoxication, is very great, since the nose and throat microflora provide a vast well of potential infection.

The method of correlating phage-susceptible strains of staphylococci (22, 46, 47) in food implicated in outbreaks with those isolated from food handlers may aid health officers in locating the source of some staphylococcus food-poisoning outbreaks and in preventing recurrent outbreaks from the same source. It is possible, with the great abundance of staphylococci in nature, that a person may not carry an enterotoxic strain one day but may carry it the next. In other words, there is always a potential danger of this type of food poisoning. On the other hand, workers with sinus infections or recurrent boils or colds should be excluded from the handling of food products.

The rapidly cured hams that are now on the market have given rise to many outbreaks of food poisoning. Many of the packers and the Meat Inspection Branch of the United States Department of Agriculture are well aware of the problem. The method involved in the heating of hams during manufacture is designed to be effective against *Trichinella* and staphylococci, so that when hams leave the packers they are safe, but they may easily become contaminated. The process of keeping ham in a warm environment for several hours, as in a kitchen, may be favorable for the growth of staphylococci and the production of enterotoxin. The important procedure in the control of food poisoning from cured-meat products is to educate the public and the retailers to the fact that such products as ham are perishable and must be kept under refrigeration. It is a well-established fact that staphylococci grow in ham without producing signs of spoilage such as abnormal odor or taste.

With the increased consumption of frozen foods, attention has been given to the potential hazard of staphylococcus food poisoning in these products. The food-poisoning staphylococci have been found to grow in low-acid foods (81): peas, corn, salmon, and shrimp. In canned string beans, spinach, and asparagus less abundant growth has occurred. In test-tube preparations of canned roast beef (82), corned beef, and potted meat, luxuriant growth takes place, and the organisms survive for at least 60 days at 22° and 37° C. when loss of moisture is prevented. Chicken à la king, creamed tuna, ham à la king, creamed salmon, turkey and noodles, and cooked shrimp have been found excellent media for the growth of food-poisoning staphylococci (83). Jones and Lockhead (69) found that, of 50 strains of micrococci isolated from frozen vegetables, 12 have produced enterotoxin. Several outbreaks (22, 84, 85) have been traced to ice cream. One outbreak has been reported from frozen fish (86).

Food-poisoning staphylococci have been found to survive freezing in creamed foods (83)—chicken à la king, ham à la king, creamed tuna, and creamed salmon, when experimentally inoculated into these products and stored at –18° C. for 9 months. In a project at the Hormel Institute (87) supported by the Navy, microörganisms were suspended in nutrient broth, milk, and liver-agar paste in 1.5 ml. of suspension containing 1×10^4 to 1×10^5 organisms per milliliter and sealed in Pyrex test tubes, 10×75 mm. A rapid freeze in an acetone dry-ice bath (—60° to —70° C.), an intermediate freeze in a solid carbon dioxide icebox (—55° C.), and a slower freeze in a deep-freeze unit with a temperature of approximately —22° C. were carried out. The freezing times were 1, 30–60, and 150 minutes, respectively. Samples were thawed in a 35° C. water bath. The statement is made that the gram-positive coccus, *S. aureus,* "appeared to be practically unaffected by any method of freezing or by any type of suspending medium." From these experimental data it is evident that viable food-poisoning staphylococci are not destroyed by freezing. Staphylococci do not produce enterotoxin at temperatures of 4°–6.°7 C. after a period of 4 weeks (74), and it is obvious that only after incubation at higher temperatures does a danger of food poisoning exist.

It is apparent that many varieties of frozen foods provide excellent nutritional conditions for the growth and enterotoxin production of food-poisoning staphylococci. Frozen foods are subject, as are all foods exposed to the atmosphere, to contamination with these microorganisms. If errors in processing occur, so that enterotoxin is formed before freezing, a potential danger from staphylococcal food poisoning arises. Furthermore, if mechanical failure of refrigeration occurs during storage, which would permit the formation of enterotoxin, the stage would be set for an outbreak of this poisoning.

In summarizing the control of staphylococcus food poisoning, several factors must be borne in mind. First, there must be sufficient contamination with an enterotoxin-producing strain of staphylococcus. Second, the food must be a good medium for the growth of the organisms and the production of enterotoxin. Third, the food must remain at or above room temperature for several hours. Of all these factors, temperature is the most practical to control.

Outbreaks have occurred where foods have been handled and placed in the refrigerator in large bulk lots, so that many hours were required for thorough chilling. Containers holding perishable items should be arranged in the refrigerator to allow good circulation of air, and the containers should hold small amounts, so that refrigeration temperatures will be reached rapidly throughout the food.

ENTEROTOXIN-PRODUCING STAPHYLOCOCCI

Some strains of staphylococci have been tested repeatedly for enterotoxin on human volunteers over a period of years and have never been found to produce it, even though the strains may produce powerful hemotoxins and lethal and dermo-necrotic toxins.[1] This has been the experience not only of the author but also of Dolman (88).

1. Hemotoxins as tested on rabbit and sheep red blood corpuscles; lethal toxins as tested by the intravenous injection of mice with filtrates; dermo-necrotic toxins as tested by the intradermal injection of rabbits with dilutions of filtrate.

The percentage of the total number of strains of staphylococci capable of producing enterotoxin is not known because, to date, no satisfactory test has been devised for differentiating the enterotoxin-from the nonenterotoxin-producing strains. Some years ago Dolman (88) worked with strains of staphylococci which produced potent hemolysins, dermotoxins, and lethal toxins but no illness in 42 volunteers on 110 occasions. A strain received from Dr. E. O. Jordan, however, yielded a filtrate, 2 ml. of which caused severe gastrointestinal disturbance in 3–9 volunteers and a lesser degree of disturbance in 4 others. On the basis of his experiments Dolman believed that the number of strains of staphylococci which produce enterotoxin is small in comparison to the total.

Stone (89) developed a cultural method for classifying staphylococci of the food-poisoning type by testing cultures in a special gelatin medium for gelatin liquefaction. Any degree of liquefaction was a positive test and indicated an enterotoxin-producing strain of staphylococcus, whereas no liquefaction indicated a negative strain. The test cultures were incubated exactly 24 hours at 37°5 C. With the use of Stone's medium, B. D. Chinn (90) established that staphylococci incriminated in food poisoning could not be differentiated by gelatin liquefaction. Chapman, Lieb, and Curcio (91) determined that the Stone reaction was positive in 70.5 per cent of typical food-poisoning staphylococci and positive in 27.6 per cent of strains with similar properties isolated from nonfood-poisoning sources. Kupchik (68) investigated the reaction to Stone's gelatin medium of 44 strains of staphylococci, many of which produced enterotoxin, and found that Stone's medium failed to exhibit any differential value. It is evident that the gelatin-liquefaction test developed by Stone is not an absolute criterion for enterotoxin production.

Stritar and Jordan (92) studied 94 strains of staphylococci from various sources. According to these workers, food-poisoning strains do not constitute a clearly marked group. By biochemical, hemolytic, or agglutinative characters there were no evidences of homogeneity. Their conclusion was that "the power to provoke food poisoning is not limited to any recognizable variety of staphylococcus."

Staphylococci grow in cured and in salted meats which prohibit the increase of spore-forming and nonspore-forming rods and in chicken containing 5 and 10 per cent salt (15). They are found numerously in wrapped minced ham and mayonnaise sandwiches purchased in drugstores (15). Hucker and Haynes (93) have shown that staphylococci will grow in concentrations of salt and sugar that are inhibitory to many bacteria. The organism is therefore not affected by salt and sugar, which are used in partially preserving certain foods. As a matter of fact, the addition of suitable concentrations of salt may serve to prevent the growth or to kill spoilage bacteria which might compete for growth with the staphylococcus.

STAPHYLOCOCCUS ENTEROTOXIN

Production of enterotoxin in synthetic media.—Surgalla (94) studied the production of staphylococcal enterotoxin in synthetic media consisting of amino acids, vitamins, inorganic salts, and glucose. He was able to detect enterotoxin in the supernatants of cultures grown in media containing from two to sixteen amino acids as the source of organic nitrogen. The amino acids arginine and cystine were present in the simplest medium. Evidence was not obtained that amino acids unessential for growth were necessary for enterotoxin production. Both growth and toxin production were reduced in the more simple media, which was attributed to the amount of available nitrogen in the media. Growth did not take place in the absence of glucose in a medium containing only three amino acids. In media containing glucose in concentrations ranging from 0.2 to 20.0 per cent, enterotoxin was demonstrated. Less enterotoxin was produced in the simple, as compared to the more complex, media.

Time and temperature for the production of enterotoxin.—It is important to know the time and temperature necessary for staphylococci to produce sufficient enterotoxin in foods that give rise to food poisoning in man. The answer to this question may be obtained through a survey of the literature. The production of enterotoxin depends, first of all, upon contamination with a food-poisoning strain of staphylococcus. The initial number of these organisms or the amount of contamination is important. If the food is heavily contaminated from the beginning, as, for example, raw milk from infected cows' udders, the organisms will be found in greater numbers in a shorter time than if the initial contamination is slight. The competition which the staphylococci may have with other bacteria present in the food is important. One type of bacteria may overgrow another. In the case of fresh meat, putrefactive bacteria might multiply so that the product would be obviously unfit for consumption and probably would not be eaten, although staphylococci might be present and produce enough enterotoxin to provoke symptoms of food poisoning. On the other hand, the food in question may not be a good medium for favorable growth of the staphylococci.

The shortest period of time to produce enterotoxin in foods is difficult to determine unless extensive experiments on human volunteers are conducted. One of the best experiments on this subject was carried out by Barber (12). This investigator found that cream which contained staphylococci was harmless when refrigerated but was toxic when left at room temperature for 5 hours. In this experiment 5 hours were sufficient for the production of enterotoxin. Whether enterotoxin could be formed in less time in the same medium and under the same temperature conditions was not tested but remains a possibility.

Hauge (39) described an outbreak among a ski party where 12 of 31 people became ill from eating potatoes mashed with raw milk. The potatoes were kept warm for $6\frac{1}{2}$ hours before serving by being wrapped in newspapers and blankets and placed in a bed. A bacteriological examination of the mashed potatoes revealed at least 16,000,-000 yellow hemolytic staphylococci per gram. The milk came from a two-cow dairy, in which one cow excreted staphylococci at the rate of 2,500 per milliliter of milk.

In two naturally occurring outbreaks the significance of time and suitable temperature is well illustrated in foods containing an enterotoxin-producing strain of staphylococcus where groups of people ate the same food items at different times. In the first outbreak reported by Tipton and Smiley (38), sliced ham was served at noon mess, and 50 cases of food poisoning occurred after 4 hours. The ham left over was ground, placed in the refrigerator, and served with scrambled eggs the following morning. One hour after breakfast 300 cases of food poisoning occurred. It is obvious that the shorter period of time from eating the implicated food to the onset of illness indicated a more potent enterotoxin, and this was further correlated with more severe symptoms. The second outbreak (95), which occurred in an upstate New York industrial plant, was traced to contaminated cream pie. The first person to become ill ate a portion about 5:30 P.M. and became ill 3½ hours later. Those people who ate the pie 9½ hours later (3:00 A.M.) became very ill within 3 hours. Examination of the pie revealed quantities of *S. aureus*. In the second outbreak, as in the first, more enterotoxin was produced, which probably followed increase in growth of the staphylococci in the food.

In the laboratory, with a favorable medium, as reported by Segalove and Dack (74), experiments were carried out to determine the shortest interval of time necessary for enterotoxin production. A good enterotoxin-producing strain of staphylococcus was used. Monkeys were fed cultures prepared as previously described. If feeding experiments were negative, monkeys were then injected intravenously with boiled filtrates, which are a more delicate test for enterotoxin. Under these experimental conditions, enterotoxin was demonstrated in a culture grown for 3 days at 18° C. and for 12 hours at 37° C. It was not produced in cultures grown for shorter periods. At 9° and 15° C. it was not produced in 7 and 3 days, respectively. At 4° and 6°7 C. it was not formed after 4 weeks. The failure of the staphylococcus to produce enterotoxin at the lower temperatures may be ascribed to poor growth. It may be concluded, therefore, that, among food-poisoning strains of staphylococci, enterotoxin production is a function of growth.

Effect of antibiotics on growth and toxin production by enterotoxic staphylococci.—Segalove (96) studied the natural resistance of 15 enterotoxic strains which were found to have a wide range of resistance to penicillin (0.05–500 units per milliliter), and 5 nonenterotoxic strains which were found relatively sensitive (0.05–0.1 unit per milliliter) to the antibiotics. The addition of penicillin to media did not inhibit enterotoxin production when good growth occurred.

The addition of antibiotics to food in order to inhibit enterotoxigenic strains of staphylococci has been considered, but scientific merit has not been established for this idea. Finland (97) makes the statement: "Staphylococci, perhaps more than any other common pathogenic bacteria, have exhibited a marked tendency to increase in resistance to available and widely used antibiotics." Evidence is given that when penicillin, chlortetracycline (aureomycin), oxytetracycline (terramycin), and erythromycin were first introduced in treating patients in hospitals, comparatively few strains of staphylococci were found which were resistant to these antibiotics. However, after a period of time, the majority of strains of staphylococci isolated from patients or hospital personnel had become resistant.

Enterotoxin produced in vivo in patients under antibiotic therapy. —A number of patients under treatment with antibiotics have been found to develop diarrhea with or without vomiting (98–103). Finland and others (103) observed a greater frequency of occurrence of gastrointestinal complications in patients treated with oxytetracycline (terramycin) than with patients treated with the same dosages of chlortetracycline (aureomycin). Diarrhea occurred in 38 per cent of the former in comparison with 18 per cent of the latter. Furthermore, when smaller individual doses were used, gastrointestinal effects were not so severe. A parallel study was undertaken with both antibiotics. With each of them, diarrhea was approximately twice as frequent among patients who received 250-mg. doses every 4 hours or 500-mg. doses every 4 or 6 hours as among those receiving 250 mg. every 6 hours. Hemolytic coagulase-positive strains of S. aureus were found as the predominant organism in fecal cultures from 27 of 38 patients treated with oxytetracycline in whom diarrhea developed. Some patients under treatment with antibiotics who developed diarrhea have alleged that their gastrointestinal symptoms were due to an item of food they had eaten, and in some instances legal action has been taken to recover damages.

The entire problem of gastrointestinal illnesses following antibiotic therapy involves the question whether or not enterotoxin is produced in vivo. Surgalla and Dack (104) tested the enterotoxigenic capacity of strains of staphylococci which had been isolated from patients in four different localities. Enterotoxin was produced from 30 out of 32 strains of staphylococci. The 2 enterotoxin-negative strains were coagulase-negative. The 2 coagulase-negative, nonenterotoxin-producing strains recovered from these cases would not exclude in vivo enterotoxin production, since it would be possible for enterotoxigenic and nonenterotoxigenic antibiotic-resistant strains to coexist in the same patient, in which case a nonenterotoxigenic strain might be recovered. In staphylococcus food poisoning, even though large numbers of viable enterotoxigenic staphylococci are ingested together with enterotoxin, there is no evidence that they multiply and produce further enterotoxin in the body. Apparently, the normal intestinal flora interferes with the growth of *S. aureus* in the intestinal tract. The bacteriological studies of Finland *et al.* (103) indicated that large numbers of staphylococci were present (sputum, urine, trachea, bronchus, throat, vomitus, abscess) in some patients under treatment with oxytetracycline. There is no reason why enterotoxin might not be produced at other sites in the bodies of these patients, which would explain the cases in which severe diarrhea occurs when the fecal cultures do not show a predominance of staphylococci. In vivo production of enterotoxin would account for the more severe pseudo-membranous enteritis and the higher death rate in such patients.

Experimental production of enterotoxin in foods.—Strains of food-poisoning staphylococci have been inoculated into foods and subsequently tested by feeding to human volunteers. These tests are outlined in Table 10.

Experiments with fresh beef liver were made by the author in conjunction with Dr. W. A. Starin at Ohio State University and are reported here in detail, since they have not appeared elsewhere in the literature. Two livers were received in a fresh state within a few hours after the animals had been slaughtered. One weighed 4,250 gm., and the other 7,050 gm. The purpose of the work was to keep the meat for the same length of time and under the same temperature conditions as in the modern butcher-shop. Before storage the livers were heavily inoculated inside and outside with a food-poisoning strain of staphylococcus which had been isolated in 1935 from tongue (105) used for sandwich filling and was known to produce potent enterotoxin. A suspension containing 3.3 billion bacteria per milliliter was injected into each liver. They were then placed in a large pan and put into an electric refrigerator. They were left in the refrigerator at a temperature of $3°3$ C. for 3 days, wrapped in three thicknesses of ordinary brown wrapping paper, and kept in a cool room ($16°6$ C.) for a period of $6\frac{1}{2}$ hours (Table 10). This procedure represented the conditions in the butcher-shop. The livers were then placed in an electric refrigerator for $6\frac{1}{2}$ hours and were later unwrapped and allowed to remain at room temperature, $23°3$ C., for 50 minutes before cooking, as might occur in the house of

TABLE 10

GROWTH AND ENTEROTOXIN PRODUCTION BY STAPHYLOCOCCI INTRODUCED INTO FOOD

FOOD	TREATMENT	INCUBA-TION (HOURS)	TEMPERA-TURE (° C.)	BACTERIAL COUNT PER GM.	KIND OF BACTERIA	HUMAN FEEDING Amount (Gm.)	HUMAN FEEDING Result
Custard cake filler (106)	None	None	....	610,000	Air contaminants (no staphylococci)	30	Negative
Custard cake filler (106)	None	22	24.4–30	High	....	30	Negative
Custard cake filler (106)	Inoculated with staphylococcus	None	....	414 million	Mostly staphylococci	30	Slightly toxic
Custard cake filler (106)	Inoculated with staphylococcus	22	24.4–30	430 million	Mostly staphylococci	5, 15	Toxic
Bread in lettuce sandwich (15)	Inoculated with staphylococcus	5, 16, 6*	37, 6, 37	1,100 million	Mostly staphylococci	63	Toxic
Home-baked ham in lettuce sandwich (15)	Inoculated with staphylococcus	5	37	30 million	Staphylococci	Ham from 1 sandwich	Negative
Home-baked ham in lettuce sandwich (15)	Inoculated with staphylococcus	5, 16, 6*	37, 6, 37	1,000 million	Staphylococci	48	Toxic
Fresh beef liver	Inoculated with staphylococcus	None	....	2.3 million	Mostly staphylococci	....	Not tested
Fresh beef liver	Inoculated with staphylococcus	72, 6.5, 6.5, 0.88*	3.3, 16.6, 5.0, 23.3	1.5 million	Staphylococci	100	Negative
Canned corn (107)	Inoculated with staphylococcus	168	37	Growth occurred	Staphylococci	30	Toxic
Canned salmon (107)	Inoculated with staphylococcus	96	37	Growth occurred	Staphylococci	90	Negative
Canned oysters (107)	Inoculated with staphylococcus	72	37	Growth occurred	Staphylococci	100	Toxic

* One test was made on this material at the end of the series of incubations.

the consumer. After this treatment, the liver was sampled for a bacteriological count and for enterotoxin. With a sterile knife, two wedge-shaped sections were cut through the long portion of the large liver, and, in addition, a similar section was cut from the smaller one. One hundred grams of this raw liver were eaten by a human volunteer who had previously been shown to be susceptible to staphylococcus enterotoxin. He experienced no ill effects. This experiment demonstrates that staphylococcus food poisoning will not occur in liver stored under the conditions of a butcher-shop, even where large numbers of enterotoxin-producing staphylococci are present. This work is in agreement with the previously mentioned experiments (74) on the time and temperature requirements for the production of enterotoxin by staphylococci.

Certain foods may support the growth of staphylococci without the production of potent enterotoxin, as, for example, canned salmon (107).[2] Other foods—meat products and custard-filled bakery goods—allow food-poisoning staphylococci to grow and to produce enterotoxin. Aside from such empirical knowledge, however, little is known of the chemical nature of enterotoxin or the chemistry of the metabolism of enterotoxic staphylococci. Staphylococcus enterotoxin is formed irregularly by some strains in veal-infusion broth in flasks incubated aerobically. The difference cannot be explained on the basis of the medium employed, because variations are observed when the same batch of medium and the same aged culture for the inoculum are used. When strains are inoculated into semisolid agar and incubated in an atmosphere containing 10–20 per cent carbon dioxide, a more potent enterotoxin is produced with greater regularity. Thus it seems reasonable that certain foods are more suitable than others for the production of enterotoxin.

During World War II dehydrated meat was produced, and the food-poisoning hazard from this product was evaluated. Segalove and Dack (108) found that an enterotoxin-producing strain of *S. aureus*, experimentally inoculated into dehydrated meat, failed to grow when the moisture content of meat samples was adjusted to 10 or 20 per cent. Growth occurred in dehydrated pork samples at

2. In unpublished experiments by Surgalla and Hite, extracts of canned salmon experimentally inoculated with enterotoxic staphylococci induced vomiting in 7 out of 51 instances when fed to monkeys.

a moisture adjusted to 30 per cent, except in one sample with a salt concentration of 4.56 per cent. In beef samples adjusted to 30 per per cent moisture, no growth occurred except for a slight increase in a sample with a salt concentration of 2.20 per cent. At 40, 50, and 60 per cent moisture, growth occurred in all samples with salt concentrations varying from 0.21 to 4.56 per cent.

Because many outbreaks of staphylococcus food poisoning have been traced to bakery goods, some workers believed that starch (109) might be of significance; others that protein (89) might be the important factor. Jordan and Burrows (109) found that bacteria of various kinds—i.e., staphylococci, streptococci, *Proteus, Escherichia coli, Bacterium aerogenes,* and *Salmonella aertrycke*—grown under suitable conditions, especially on starch medium, were capable of producing a substance which caused gastrointestinal reactions in monkeys. By successive transfers on starch media, they further succeeded in restoring the enterotoxic property to strains which had lost the ability to produce the substance. They claimed that bacteria which had never possessed this characteristic could produce the toxic material when grown on starch medium. Other workers (110) have not been able to confirm the work of Jordan and Burrows. Filtrates were prepared from 12 different kinds of bacteria, which had been grown in media with and without starch. The starch-culture filtrate and the corresponding control filtrate without starch were fed in triplicate to monkeys. These animals were observed continuously for a period of 5 hours and at intervals of 8, 12, and 24 hours after feeding, but no symptoms of food poisoning were observed. At the conclusion of these experiments, similarly prepared filtrates from a known food-poisoning staphylococcus strain were fed. Four of the 6 animals vomited and showed typical symptoms of food poisoning.

PURIFICATION OF ENTEROTOXIN

Dialysis.—Several attempts have been made to purify enterotoxin, but in most cases very little purification has been attained. The effectiveness of certain reagents for concentration of the toxin in bacterial filtrates was explored and reported. Jordan and Burrows (111) found that the active principle of enterotoxin was not readily dialyzable. Other investigators have confirmed this observation.

Ammonium sulphate precipitation.—It was demonstrated by Davison and Dack (112) that enterotoxin was consistently "salted out" from saturated solutions of ammonium sulphate but not from half-saturated solutions. Hammon (70) reported that the other toxins of staphylococci are precipitated from 75 per cent saturated ammonium sulphate solutions, whereas the enterotoxin remained in solution. Bergdoll, Kadavy, Surgalla, and Dack (113) reported that they were able to precipitate some enterotoxin from 50 per cent saturated ammonium sulphate solutions, most of it from 75 per cent saturated solutions, and all of it from saturated solutions. The percentage of the enterotoxin that could be precipitated from 75 per cent saturated solutions appeared to be dependent upon the amount of enterotoxin present in the original solutions.

Ethanol precipitation.—Davison and Dack (112) attempted to precipitate enterotoxin from 76 per cent ethanol solutions at pH 6.8, 7.2, and 8.0. The mixtures were refrigerated overnight before the precipitates were removed. Although conditions of pH, time, temperature, etc., were controlled, the results obtained at one time were not always duplicated at another. Hammon was able to precipitate enterotoxin repeatedly from 63 per cent ethanol solutions. The mixture was allowed to stand at 2° C. for 24–48 hours before the precipitate was removed by centrifugation. Bergdoll and co-workers (113) were able to precipitate enterotoxin from 40 per cent ethanol at −5° to −10° C. The toxin solution was adjusted to pH 6.0 and an ionic strength of 0.1 before the ethanol was added. The mixture was allowed to stand overnight before the precipitate was removed by filtration or centrifugation. These conditions insured against the possible inactivation of the toxin by ethanol.

Acid precipitation.—Bergdoll and associates (113, 114) succeeded in recovering much of the enterotoxin from bacterial filtrates by acid precipitation. This was accomplished by adjusting the pH of the bacterial filtrates to 3.5 with hydrochloric or phosphoric acid and removing the precipitate by filtration through a layer of filter aid, such as Hyflo Super Cel. Less enterotoxin was recovered when the precipitate was removed by centrifugation. The fact that enterotoxin could be recovered by this procedure was apparently due to adsorption of the toxin (1) on the impurities that were precipitated and (2) on the filter aid.

Chromatography.—Various chromatographic procedures have

been studied in an attempt to purify the enterotoxin. A ten to twenty fold purification of the toxin present in partially purified preparations was accomplished by chromatographing on the filter aid, Hyflo Super Cel (115). The toxin was adsorbed from a citrate-phosphate buffer solution of pH 6.35 and an ionic strength of 0.02 and eluted from the Hyflo Super Cel with a citrate-phosphate buffer solution of pH 7.8 and an ionic strength of 0.12. Similar results were obtained with alumina as the adsorbent. In this case the toxin was adsorbed from a 0.02 M phosphate buffer solution of pH 6.35 and eluted with a 0.1 M disodium phosphate solution. Enterotoxin can also be chromatographed on the cation-exchange resin, Amberlite XF-64 (IRC-50). The enterotoxin was quantitatively adsorbed from a 0.02 M phosphate buffer solution of pH 6.2 and eluted with a 0.2 M phosphate buffer solution of pH 6.2. It has not been possible to eliminate all the impurities by these chromatographic procedures.

Electrophoresis.—Electrophoresis with starch as a supporting medium has been employed in the purification of enterotoxin. Partially purified enterotoxin could be separated into two fractions by this technique when a 0.05 M phosphate buffer solution at pH 6.0 was used to prepare the starch bed. At this pH the enterotoxin moved toward the cathode and was present in the fraction that contained 20 per cent of the nitrogen present in the starting material. The Oudin immunological technique showed that at least three of the major antigens present in the original sample were removed with the nontoxic fraction.

Heavy metals.—The use of heavy metals (zinc) for the precipitation of enterotoxin has been investigated (114). The toxin in bacterial filtrates was precipitated at pH 6.8 when sufficient zinc acetate was added to bring the zinc concentration to 0.02 M. Large amounts of contaminating materials were also precipitated by this reagent.

Purification schemes.—The procedures outlined here have been combined in various ways in attempts to obtain pure enterotoxin. Hammon's first step in his attempt to purify enterotoxin was to remove some of the impurities by precipitating them from 75 per cent saturated ammonium sulphate solutions. After the supernatant fluid was dialyzed to remove the sulphate, the enterotoxin was precipitated by the addition of 2 volumes of 95 per cent ethanol. Positive reactions were obtained when 2–6.5 ml. of the purified toxin solutions were injected intravenously into cats. The total solids in one preparation were found to be 1.8 mg/ml.

Bergdoll (114) precipitated the toxin from bacterial filtrates with phosphoric acid at pH 3.5 and removed the precipitate by filtration through Hyflo Super Cel. The dissolved precipitate was chromatographed on alumina, with phosphate buffer as the eluting agent. The eluate was precipitated from 40 per cent ethanol at $-7°$ to $-10°$ C. The dialyzed, lyophilized material gave positive reactions in cats when 0.005–0.01 mg. was injected (boiled for 30 minutes) and in monkeys when 0.25 mg. was injected by stomach tube. It was possible to purify this material another two- to fourfold by chromatographing on the cation-exchange resin, XE-64, or another fivefold by electrophoresis with starch as the supporting medium.

PROPERTIES OF ENTEROTOXIN

Potency.—All the toxin preparations that have been obtained contained a very small percentage of enterotoxin. Bergdoll, who found the most potent preparation, estimated that the toxin content of the material did not exceed 5 per cent. He further speculated that vomiting in monkeys might be obtained with as little as 0.005 mg. of pure toxin injected orally or in cats with as little as 0.0002 mg. injected intraperitoneally. It was recognized that the results obtained from the determination of the properties of a compound present in such small amounts can be misleading. This may account for the differences of opinion about the chemical nature of the enterotoxin.

Molecular size.—The molecular weight of enterotoxin cannot be determined until pure toxin is available, but an upper and lower limit may be estimated from present information. Davison (107) states that enterotoxin will pass through a collodion membrane of $3:5$ mμ pore size. Since a particle passing a small membrane is one-third to one-half the size of the pore, according to Elford (116), the upper limit of molecular size of the enterotoxin is about 1.7 mμ. This would indicate a maximum molecular weight of less than 15,-000–20,000. A minimum molecular weight of 8,000–10,000 is indicated from the fact that enterotoxin will not pass through Visking cellulose sausage casing.

Solubility.—Enterotoxin is soluble in water and in dilute salt solutions. It is insoluble in organic solvents, such as ether (70) and chloroform (112). Its solubility in ethanol and more concentrated salt solutions has already been discussed.

Response to proteolytic enzymes.—Minett (65) found that entero-toxin was resistant to rennet but was destroyed by trypsin. Davison reported that it was destroyed by pepsin. Hammon stated that it was resistant to both trypsin and pepsin. Bergdoll *et al.* (113, 114) have obtained variable results with trypsin. Crude trypsin preparations appeared to inactivate the enterotoxin, whereas in the first experiments with crystalline trypsin no inactivation was apparent. Further experimentation with crystalline trypsin failed to resolve this problem satisfactorily, as in most cases only partial inactivation was obtained. Further studies must be made before any definite conclusions can be drawn, but the fact that partial inactivation was obtained might indicate a protein-type substance.

Chemical nature.—Hammon was unable to detect any nitrogen in his enterotoxin preparations but demonstrated the presence of a reducing carbohydrate substance. He stated that it seemed probable that the active substance was a large, complex, carbohydrate molecule.

Bergdoll's preparation (114) contained 15 per cent nitrogen, which was present in the form of amino acids. A positive test for protein was obtained by both the Biuret test and Lowry's modification of the Folin method (117). The Molisch test for carbohydrate indicated as little as 1 per cent carbohydrate. These investigators have tentatively concluded that enterotoxin is a protein or a derivative thereof. Since the enterotoxin content of their preparations was too small for the chemical identification tests to be reliable, they based their conclusions on the following: (1) enterotoxin is adsorbed by cation-exchange resins; (2) it is precipitated by zinc; (3) electrophoresis indicates that enterotoxin has an isoelectric point; (4) it is partially inactivated by trypsin; (5) it can be concentrated with methods primarily useful in the concentration of proteins; and (6) it is partially inactivated by heat.

STABILITY OF ENTEROTOXIN

Formalin.—Filtrates of staphylococci were treated with formalin, so that a final concentration of 0.3 per cent was attained. After incubation for 36 or 48 hours at 37° C., the formalinized filtrates produced vomiting in kittens. In another experiment, however, enterotoxin was inactivated by 0.3 per cent formalin after 10 days at 37° C. (65).

Chlorine.—Chlorine in unplatable amounts is not effective in destroying enterotoxin. Thus 0.1 ml. of 0.0915 per cent chlorine solution was added to 5 ml. of staphylococcus filtrate containing enterotoxin and allowed to stand for 3 minutes at room temperature, after which the chlorinated filtrate was added to $\frac{1}{2}$ pint of milk and swallowed by a human volunteer. Typical symptoms occurred in $5\frac{1}{4}$ hours (118).

pH.—There have been some discrepancies in the literature regarding the effect of acids on enterotoxin. Minett (65) treated boiled filtrate with hydrochloric acid to bring the pH to 5.0 and incubated the filtrate at room temperature and also at 37° C. In one case enterotoxin did not resist 1 week at room temperature. Hammon lowered the pH of a culture of enterotoxin to 4.5 and found active enterotoxin in the supernatant fluid after an incubation of 24 hours at 37° C. Similar treatment with sodium hydroxide to bring the filtrate to a pH of 8.0 or 8.2 appeared to have no deleterious effect. Bergdoll and workers (113) found no inactivation of enterotoxin when it was held at pH 3.5 for 22 hours at 4° C. In another experiment enterotoxin samples were held in solution at pH 3, 8, 10, and 12 for 4 hours at room temperature. Enterotoxin was still present in all samples except the one held at pH 12 (114).

Storage.—Staphylococcus filtrates containing enterotoxin have been demonstrated toxic after storage for as long as 67 days in an electric refrigerator (118). The tests were made by feeding human volunteers 5-ml. portions of filtrates from veal-infusion broth cultures grown in a normal atmosphere. In view of the individual differences in susceptibility in human volunteers, it is uncertain whether a slight loss of potency might not have occurred during the storage period. Bergdoll demonstrated that partially purified enterotoxin can be stored in the dry state at 37° C. for at least 8 months without apparent loss in toxicity.

Heat.—Enterotoxin which was produced by growing a strain of staphylococcus in beef-infusion broth incubated aerobically was boiled for 30 minutes. When 2 and 10 ml. were fed, respectively, to

2 human volunteers, typical symptoms occurred in both (118). Blood was present in the vomitus and stools of the individual receiving 10 ml. Subsequently, the effect of heat on enterotoxin (114) was studied in monkeys. Filtrates were prepared from 3-day cultures grown on semisolid veal-infusion agar in an environment of 20 per cent carbon dioxide. The medium was strained through gauze, and the fluid which was expressed was centrifugalized to remove most of the organisms and then passed through a Berkefeld "N" filter. This filtrate was subjected to the temperatures in Table 11 and injected intravenously into monkeys in doses of 0.2, 0.5, and 1.0

TABLE 11

HEAT STABILITY OF STAPHYLOCOCCUS ENTEROTOXIN

Treatment	No. Monkeys	No. Positive	Per Cent Positive
Boiled 20 min..............	15	4	27
Boiled 30 min..............	21	7	33
Boiled 60 min..............	14	2	14
Autoclaved 20 min. (120° C., 15 lb. pressure)..........	14	1	7

ml. per kilogram of body weight. It is evident from the results (Table 11) that enterotoxin is extremely heat-resistant but gradually loses its potency with prolonged boiling or autoclaving. The rate of destruction is difficult to quantitate, however, since susceptibility to the enterotoxin in both man and animals varies and the latter may develop a tolerance to the enterotoxin.

Drysdale (55) describes an outbreak of staphylococcous food poisoning caused by drinking boiled milk. All 30 members of a club who had been served coffee with boiled milk bought from an Arab goatherd became ill. Four members served tea with cow's milk obtained from a model dairy were not affected. The Arab goat's milk was boiled before being served but was not treated otherwise. All 30 who became ill developed symptoms within 1 hour, and a large proportion of the patients had to be admitted to a hospital. Some individuals were in a state of collapse. Five households in Khartoum City were also affected, which brought the casualties to 75 in all. The boiled milk was examined bacteriologically, and no growth of

S. aureus or any other significant organism was found. Coagulase-positive *S. aureus* was found in the unboiled, implicated milk. A portion of the boiled milk fed to a monkey (*Cercopithecus aethiops*) produced vomiting and diarrhea after 1 hour. No metallic or other gastrointestinal poisons were found in the milk by a government analyst. The Arab contractor's milk supply was found to be derived principally from a herd of goats, one of which was found to have mastitis. Strains of staphylococci from the unboiled milk and the infected goat were typed by Dr. Allison at the Central Public Health Laboratory at Colindale, England, and both were found to be of the same phage type. Millar and Pownall (119) report a case of staphylococcus food poisoning traceable to meat and gravy prepared by a man who had burned his fingers and the blisters became infected with *S. aureus*. (The meat and gravy were eaten hot almost immediately after cooking.) Greene (120) reports an outbreak traceable to pasteurized milk. Nevot and others (121) describe one due to pork sausage and mention that the cooking to which the product is subjected is insufficient to destroy toxic properties. Hauge (39) cites outbreaks demonstrating the effectiveness of pasteurization in destroying staphylococci but not preformed enterotoxin. Surgalla and Dack (122) found that fresh pork shoulder roasts experimentally inoculated with a culture of staphylococcus containing enterotoxin and cooked in hot fat for $2\frac{2}{3}$ hours did not affect human volunteers who ate them. From the evidence cited it is obvious that enterotoxin in certain foods is relatively heat-stable. Until a reliable assay method for enterotoxin becomes available, it will be difficult to evaluate the heat stability of enterotoxin in a variety of food products. The evidence indicates that every effort should be made to prevent the formation of enterotoxin before the food is processed or consumed.

Bergdoll *et al.* (113) held partially purified enterotoxin preparations in solution at pH 6.0 and 7.5 at 100° C. for 30 minutes before oral injection into monkeys. The results indicated at least a 95 per cent inactivation of the enterotoxin. When another partially purified enterotoxin sample was boiled for 30 minutes and injected intraperitoneally into cats, positive reactions were obtained with as little as 0.016 mg. of the sample (114). It was impossible to determine whether any inactivation of the toxin occurred in this experiment, since in any case it was necessary to heat the enterotoxin sample to destroy the other toxins present. From the data available, however, it would appear that heat changes the toxin and makes it ineffective for oral injection into monkeys but not for intraperitoneal or intravenous injection into cats or monkeys.

Antigenicity.—Surgalla, Bergdoll, and Dack have demonstrated that enterotoxin can be completely neutralized by antiserums produced in the rabbit (123), monkey, and horse (124) by using Freund adjuvants. The rabbits and monkeys were immunized with partially purified toxin by various routes, the horse subcutaneously. The enterotoxin was assayed by the monkey-feeding test. Relatively large amounts of some of these antiserums were necessary to neutralize the toxin completely.

Dolman, Wilson, and Cockcroft (66) have reported that enterotoxin was antigenic, since kittens given several spaced injections of enterotoxic filtrate became resistant and blood serum from one kitten neutralized the enterotoxic properties of an equal volume of potent filtrate to such an extent that the mixture proved innocuous when injected into a normal kitten. Dack (63) found that antiserum, when mixed with filtrates containing enterotoxic substances and injected intraperitoneally into kittens, prevented vomiting, but when the same mixture was injected intracardially into kittens or intravenously into monkeys, food-poisoning symptoms occurred. When normal kitten blood was added to a mixture of enterotoxic filtrate and antiserum and then injected intraperitoneally into normal kittens, protection was not assured. Furthermore, monkeys immunized with a filtrate containing enterotoxin were protected against enterotoxin given by the oral route but not against enterotoxin given intravenously. Our present knowledge indicates that complete neutralization of the toxin would have occurred if sufficient antitoxin had been used. One would expect to obtain weak antisera when crude toxin is used for immunization because only a very small percentage of the crude material is actually toxin. When partially purified preparations are used for immunization, more potent antisera are obtained (124).

It has not been demonstrated that antitoxin is produced in animals that receive the toxin by mouth, but it is assumed that the developed resistance in these animals to the toxin is due to the formation of antitoxin. In experiments (49) in which 4 human subjects were fed gradually increasing doses of staphylococcus filtrates from veal-in-fusion broth cultures grown in a normal atmosphere in amounts reaching 25–32 ml., a tolerance appeared to develop to the entero-toxin. The tolerance was not high; and at the conclusion of the ex-periment another more potent filtrate prepared from the same strain of staphylococcus, when fed to 3 of the 4 volunteers, produced ill-ness in 2. Serum from "immunized" men (49) and rabbits did not protect monkeys or rabbits when mixed with potent filtrate and in-jected intravenously, nor did the serum protect a human volunteer who swallowed it mixed with potent filtrate. As only minute quanti-ties of enterotoxin are necessary to cause illness, it is probable that the amounts reaching the vascular system following oral injection are so small that the buildup of antitoxin is very slow and erratic. Eventually, however, the antitoxin level should reach a point suf-ficient to neutralize the small amounts of toxin entering the circula-tion from the digestive tract but not sufficient to neutralize the rela-tively larger amounts of toxin introduced parenterally. These con-siderations substantiate the following statement by Barber (12) relative to immunity:

Persons who had used the milk continuously had apparently developed some tolerance to the toxin. Two children of the family had used the milk regularly, but never had attacks. The adults had occasional light attacks, or, in one or two cases, some chronic intestinal trouble. In my own case, 4 acute attacks, 3 of them severe, afforded no protection against a subsequent fifth dose. Visitors at the farm and Filipino employees who used the milk less regularly showed most severe attacks. Since the discontinuance of the use of raw milk from this cow, all trouble has ceased.

The agar diffusion technique of Oudin has been used to follow purification of enterotoxin with the hope of eventually identifying the toxin with one of the precipitate bands (125). By quantitative application of the technique, approximate equivalence ratios were determined for the antigens giving visible precipitates (123).

Hemolytic, dermo-necrotic, and lethal toxins are the same anti-genically for different strains and may be neutralized by a common antitoxin. This may not be true for enterotoxin, however, since Sur-galla *et al.* (124) have obtained evidence that indicates enterotoxin from one strain of staphylococcus may not be completely neutralized by antiserum obtained from toxin preparations from another strain. This would corroborate the monkey-feeding observations that monkeys resistant to enterotoxin from one strain of staphylococcus may not be resistant to the enterotoxin from other strains (64).

MODE OF ACTION OF ENTEROTOXIN

The mode of action of the staphylococcal enterotoxin has not been conclusively demonstrated. Bayliss (126) attempted to localize the site of action of enterotoxin by the use of various surgical procedures and drugs. The parenteral administration of enterotoxic preparations produced emesis following the removal of the celiac ganglion, removal of the stomach, severance of the spinal cord at the level of the second or lower thoracic vertebra, or unilateral vagotomy. Mild retching movements and rarely emesis occurred when enterotoxin was injected following transection of the spinal cord at the level of the seventh cervical vertebra, abdominal evisceration, or sectioning of both vagus nerves. Vomiting did not occur after ablation of the region of the floor of the fourth ventricle or after decerebration by transection of the brain between the anterior border of the pons and the posterior border of the hypothalmus. Morphine inhibited, ergotoxine inhibited or delayed, whereas atropine had little or no effect on emesis due to the injection of enterotoxin. On the basis of his findings, Bayliss concluded that the staphylococcal enterotoxin produced emesis by acting on the peripheral sensory structures of the viscera, especially the small intestine, the impulses passing to the central nervous system mainly through the vagus nerves. The brain centers anterior to the medulla were also considered as influencing the vomiting mechanism.

Borison and Wang (127) reviewing the work of Bayliss (126), point out that the only basis for a peripheral receptor site for the action of enterotoxin was the markedly reduced sensitivity of cats to enterotoxin as a consequence of double vagotomy. Although there are objections to the use of acute animal preparations for investigations of this type, these authors considered it noteworthy that not a single instance of vomiting occurred in 7 animals that had been decerebrated. They suggested the possibility that the site of emetic action of enterotoxin is situated in the forebrain.

The work of Bayliss may possibly be open to another objection. The boiled enterotoxic filtrates used in the experiments did not provoke vomiting in the cats, even when fed up to a dosage of 30 ml.

per kilogram of body weight, although emesis occurred when 1–2 ml. per kilogram were given intraperitoneally, intravenously, or intracardially. Although cats seem to be less sensitive to the emetic action of enterotoxin given orally as compared to intraperitoneal or intravenous injection, more controls would seem advisable, since the reliability of intraperitoneal administration of boiled staphylococcal filtrates as a specific means of detecting enterotoxin has not been universally accepted.

Bayliss (126) observed no consistent differences when isolated strips of cat or rabbit intestine suspended in Ringer's solution were treated with enterotoxic and nonenterotoxic filtrates. However, Richmond, Reed, Shaughnessy, and Michael (128) suggested that the increased tonus of isolated segments of rabbit intestine when treated with filtrates from an enterotoxic strain of staphylococcus might be similar to the enterospasm experienced in food poisoning. Anderson (129) obtained a characteristic increase in tone of isolated segments of small intestines of the rabbit with all twelve of the food-poisoning strains tested. On the other hand, attempts to confirm these observations by using the partially purified enterotoxin prepared by Surgalla, Bergdoll, and Dack in the author's laboratories have indicated that the response studied is not due to enterotoxin (125). Enterotoxin did not affect the reaction of isolated intestinal or uterine strips to adrenalin. Similarly, it does not have any influence on the in vitro peristalsis of isolated intestinal segments (Trendelenburg's method) and does not relieve the inhibition of peristalsis produced by hexamethonium (130).

The application of filtrates derived from enterotoxigenic staphylococcus strains to the nerve portion of a frog sciatic nerve–gastrocnemius muscle preparation evoked contraction of the muscle. A possible relationship between this neurotoxic effect of the filtrates and enterotoxin was suggested by Holtman and Peterson (131). This reaction was found not to be caused by enterotoxin when tested with partially purified enterotoxin (130). Enterotoxin did not show any significant effect on the isolated phrenic nerve–diaphragm muscle preparations of the rat. The conduction of the nerve impulse was not affected when the sciatic and phrenic nerves of the cat were treated similarly.

The possible effects of enterotoxin on various heart preparations have been studied. The frog heart (Straub preparation), isolated rabbit auricle, and embryonic chick hearts have shown no response which could be attributed to enterotoxin.

Since increased salivation is a frequent symptom of the staphylococcal food-poisoning syndrome, salivation of cats has been studied. When cats under chloralose anesthesia are salivating at a constant rate under carbachol stimulation, the intravenous injection of enterotoxin preparations frequently increases the salivation; however, this response is not very sensitive (130).

Various enzymatic systems have been used in the attempt to find the mode of action of enterotoxin. Enterotoxin does not affect glycolysis. The phosphorus-oxygen uptake ratio by rat liver mitochondria was studied, but the toxicity of the nonenterotoxic control preparations made this study difficult to interpret (130). Apyrase activity can be shown in some of the partially purified enterotoxins (132), but the highest activity has been found in a preparation of very low enterotoxicity. Enterotoxin does not affect cholinesterase or the acetylation mechanism.

REFERENCES

1. PASTEUR, L. Bull. Acad. méd., Paris, 9:447, 1880.
2. ROSENBACH, F. J. Mikroorganism bei d. Wundinfektionskrankheiten. Wiesbaden, 1884.
3. Edinburgh M. & Surg. J., 34:215, 1830.
4. BUCKENHAM, JOHN. Lancet, 2:297, 1862.
5. MACKEY, EDWARD. Brit. M. J., 1:533, 1873.
6. LEFFMANN, H. M. Bull., 1:68, 1879.
7. VAUGHAN, V. C. Pub. Health Papers & Rep., Am. Pub. Health A., 10:241–45, 1884.
8. STERNBERG, G. M. 13th ann. rep., secretary, State Board of Health, State of Michigan, pp. 218–26, 1885.
9. ———. A textbook of bacteriology, p. 148. 2d rev. ed. Baltimore: William Wood & Co., 1901.
10. Bull. Acad. roy. de méd. de Belgique, 4th ser., 8:496, 1894.
11. OWEN, ROBERT W. G. Physician & Surgeon, 29:289, 1907.
12. BARBER, M. A. Philippine J. Sc., sec. B, 9:515–19, 1914.
13. BAERTHLEIN, KARL. Ueber ausgedehnte Wurstvergiftungen, bedingt durch Bacillus proteus vulgaris. München. med. Wchnschr., 69:155–56, 1922.
14. DACK, G. M., CARY, W. E., WOOLPERT, O., and WIGGERS, H. J. Prevent. Med. 4:167–75, 1930.
15. KELLY, FLORENE C., and DACK, G. M. Am. J. Pub. Health, 26:1077–82, 1936.

16. SLOCUM, G. G., and LINDEN, B. A. Am. J. Pub. Health, **29**:1326-30, 1939.
17. CAUDILL, F. W., and HUMPHREY, E. C. Kentucky M. J., **37**:373-74, 1939.
18. KODAMA, T., HATA, M., and SIBUYA, Y. Kitasato Arch. Exper. Med., Japan, **17**:115-26, 1940.
19. TIMMERMAN, W. A. Nederl. tijdschr. geneesk., **81**:4443-47, 1937; abstr., J.A.M.A., **109**:1590, 1937.
20. WEED, L. A., MICHAEL, A. C., and HARGER, R. N. Am. J. Pub. Health, **33**:1314-18, 1943.
21. ODDY, J. G., and CLEGG, H. W. Brit. M. J., **1**:442, 1947.
22. WILLIAMS, G. C., SWIFT, S., VOLLUM, R. L., and WILSON, G. S. Month. Bull. Min. Health, **5**:17-25, 1946.
23. LUMSDEN, L. L., NAU, C. A., and STEAD, F. M. Pub. Health Rep., **58**:1497-1507, 1943.
24. DOYLE, H. S. Canad. J. Pub. Health, **37**:65-68, 1946.
25. DE LAY, P. D. Bull. U.S. Army M. Dept., Washington, D.C., **72**:71-73, 1944.
26. WETHINGTON, MARY C., and FABIAN, F. W. Food Res., **15**:125-34, 1950.
27. Pub. Health Rep., **56**:2277-84, 1941.
28. COUGHLIN, F. E., and JOHNSON, BASCOM. Am. J. Pub. Health, **31**:245-50, 1941.
29. FEIG, MILTON. Am. J. Pub. Health, **40**:1372-94, 1950.
30. DAUER, C. C. Pub. Health Rep., **67**:1089-95, 1952.
31. ———. *Ibid.*, **68**:696-702, 1953.
32. ———. *Ibid.*, **69**:538-45, 1954.
33. Chemistry & Industry, pp. 54-55, February 17, 1945.
34. Month. Bull. Min. Health, **9**:149, 1950.
35. ———. *Ibid.*, p. 255.
36. ———. *Ibid.*, **10**:228, 1951.
37. ———. *Ibid.*, **13**:12, 1954.
38. U.S. Nav. M. Bull., **41**:565-73, 1943.
39. HAUGE, STEINAR. Nord. vet. med., **3**:931-56, 1951.
40. PLASTRIDGE, W. N., ANDERSON, E. O., WILLIAMS, L. F., and WEIRETHER, F. J. Storrs Agr. Exper. Stat., Connecticut State College, Bull. 231, January, 1939.
41. LITTLE, R. B., and PLASTRIDGE, W. N. Bovine mastitis. New York: McGraw-Hill Book Co., 1946.
42. SLANETZ, L. W., and BARTLEY, CLARA H. J. Infect. Dis., **92**:139-51, 1953.
43. BURNET, F. M., and LUSH, D. J. Path. & Bact., **40**:455-69, 1935.
44. FISK, ROY T. J. Infect. Dis., **71**:153-60, 161-65, 1942.
45. BLAIR, J. E., and CARR, M. J. Infect. Dis., **93**:1-13, 1953.
46. WILSON, G. S., and ATKINSON, J. D. Lancet, **248**:647, 1945.
47. MCCLURE, W. B., and MILLER, A. M. Canad. M. A. J., **55**:36-39, 1946.
48. DENISON, G. A. Am. J. Pub. Health, **26**:1168-75, 1936.
49. DACK, G. M., JORDAN, EDWIN O., and WOOLPERT, ORAM. J. Prevent. Med., **5**:151-59, 1931.

50. McBurney, Ralph. J.A.M.A., **100**:1999–2001, 1933.
51. Dolman, C. E. Canad. Pub. Health J., **27**:494–97, 1936.
52. Roberts, James, Deadman, W. J., and Elliott, F. J. Canad. Pub. Health J., **29**:325–28, 1938.
53. Cogswell, W. F., Kilbourne, B. R., and Kuhns, E. Canad. Pub. Health J., **29**:333–36, 1938.
54. Roberts, James. Canad. Pub. Health J., **30**:592, 1939.
55. Drysdale, A. Trop. Med., **53**:12–14, 1950.
56. Evans, James B. J. Bact., **55**:793–800, 1948.
57. Evans, James B., and Niven, C. F., Jr. J. Bact., **59**:545–50, 1950.
58. Evans, James B., Buettner, L. G., and Niven, C. F., Jr. J. Bact., **60**:481–84, 1950.
59. Woolpert, Oram C., and Dack, G. M. J. Infect. Dis., **52**:6–19, 1933.
60. Favorite, Grant O., and Hammon, William McD. J. Bact., **41**: 305–16, 1941.
61. Surgalla, M. J., Kadavy, J. L., Bergdoll, M. S., and Dack, G. M. J. Infect. Dis., **89**:180–84, 1951.
62. Jordan, Edwin O., and McBroom, Josephine. Proc. Soc. Exper. Biol. & Med., **29**:161–62, 1931.
63. Davison, Ellen, Dack, G. M., and Cary, W. E. J. Infect. Dis., **62**: 219–23, 1938.
64. Surgalla, M. J., Bergdoll, M. S., and Dack, G. M. J. Lab. & Clin. Med., **41**:782–88, 1953.
65. Minett, F. C. J. Hyg., **38**:623–37, 1938.
66. Dolman, C. E., Wilson, R. J., and Cockcroft, W. H. Canad. Pub. Health J., **27**:489–93, 1936.
67. Surgalla, Michael J., and Hite, K. Eileen. J. Infect. Dis., **76**:78–82, 1945.
68. Kupchik, George J. J. Infect. Dis., **61**:320–24, 1937.
69. Rigdon, R. H. Proc. Soc. Exper. Biol. & Med., **38**:82–84, 1938.
    Jones, A. H., and Lockhead, A. G. Food Res., **4**:203–16, 1939.
    Singer, A., and Hogan, W. A. J. Bact., **41**:74–75, 1941.
70. Am. J. Pub. Health, **31**:1191–98, 1941.
71. Robinton, Elizabeth D. Proc. Soc. Exper. Biol. & Med., **72**:265–66, 1949.
72. ———. Yale J. Biol. & Med., **23**:94–98, 1950.
73. Eddy, Cornelia A. Proc. Soc. Exper. Biol. & Med., **78**:131–34, 1951.
74. Segalove, Milton, and Dack, G. M. Food Res., **6**:127–33, 1941.
75. Stritar, Joseph, Dack, G. M., and Jungewaelter, Frank G. Food Res., **1**:237–46, 1936.
76. Baltimore Health News, **13**:144–46, 1936–37.
77. Gilcreas, F. W., and Coleman, Marion B. Am. J. Pub. Health, **31**: 956–58, 1941.
78. Castellani, A. G. Appl. Microbiol., **1**:195–99, 1953.
79. American Institute of Baking. Bull. No. 79, May, 1954.
80. Roberts, J., and Wilson, R. J. Canad. Pub. Health J., **30**:590–98, 1939.
81. Segalove, Milton, Davison, Ellen, and Dack, G. M. Food Res., **8**:54–57, 1943.

82. SURGALLA, MICHAEL, and DACK, G. M. Food Res., **10**:108–13, 1945.
83. PHILLIPS, A. W., JR., and PROCTOR, B. E. J. Bact., **54**:49, 1947.
84. McCASTLINE, W. B., THOMPSON, R., and ISAACS, M. L. J. Bact., **33**: 50–51, 1937.
85. Health News, New York State Dept. Health, **17**:104, 1940.
86. TANNER, F. W. Microbiology of foods, p. 30. 2d ed. Champaign, Ill.: Garrard Press, 1944.
87. ULRICH, J., and HALVORSON, H. O. Ann. Rep., pp. 44–46. Hormel Inst., Univ. Minnesota, 1946–47.
88. DOLMAN, C. E. J. Infect. Dis., **55**:172–83, 1934.
89. STONE, R. V. Proc. Soc. Exper. Biol. & Med., **33**:185–87, 1935.
90. CHINN, BEN D., Food Res., **1**:513–16, 1936.
91. CHAPMAN, GEORGE H., LIEB, CLARENCE W., and CURCIO, LILLIAN G. Food Res., **2**:349–67, 1937.
92. STRITAR, J., and JORDAN, E. O. J. Infect. Dis., **56**:1–7, 1935.
93. HUCKER, G. J., and HAYNES, W. C. Am. J. Pub. Health, **27**:590–94, 1937.
94. SURGALLA, MICHAEL J. J. Infect. Dis., **81**:97–111, 1947.
95. J.A.M.A., **119**:1516, 1942.
96. SEGALOVE, MILTON. J. Infect. Dis., **81**:228–43, 1947.
97. FINLAND, MAXWELL. Bull. New York Acad. Med., **30**:478–79, 1954.
98. JACKSON, G. G., and FINLAND, M. Ann. Int. Med., **35**:1175, 1951.
99. DEARING, WILLIAM H., and HEILMAN, FORDYCE R. Proc. Staff Meet. Mayo Clin., **28**:121–34, 1953.
100. FAIRLIE, CHESTER W., and KENDALL, RALPH E. J.A.M.A., **153**:90–94, 1953.
101. TERPLAN, K., PAINE, J. R., SHEFFER, J., EGAN, R., and LANSKY, H. Gastroenterology, **24**:476–509, 1953.
102. CRAMER, R., and ROSSI, E. Helvet. paediat. acta, **8**:544–60, 1953; abstr., J.A.M.A., Vol. **155**, June 19, 1954.
103. FINLAND, MAXWELL, GRIGSBY, MARGARET E., and HAIGHT, THOMAS H. A.M.A. Arch. Int. Med., **93**:23–43, 1954.
104. SURGALLA, MICHAEL J., and DACK, GAIL M. J.A.M.A., **158**:649–50, 1955.
105. DACK, G. M., BOWMAN, GEORGE W., and HARGER, R. N. J.A.M.A., **105**:1598–99, 1935.
106. DACK, G. M., WOOLPERT, ORAM, NOBLE, ISABEL, and HALLIDAY, EVELYN G. J. Prevent. Med., **5**:391–400, 1931.
107. DAVISON, E. Doctoral diss., University of Chicago, 1940.
108. SEGALOVE, MILTON, and DACK, G. M. Food Res., **16**:118–25, 1951.
109. JORDAN, EDWIN O., and BURROWS, WILLIAM. J. Infect. Dis., **57**:121–28, 1935.
110. HUNTER, FRANK R., and DACK, G. M. J. Infect. Dis., **63**:346–47, 1938.
111. JORDAN, EDWIN O., and BURROWS, WILLIAM. Proc. Soc. Exper. Biol. & Med., **30**:448–49, 1933.
112. DAVISON, ELLEN, and DACK, G. M. J. Infect. Dis., **64**:302–6, 1939.
113. BERGDOLL, M. S., KADAVY, J. L., SURGALLA, M. J., and DACK, G. M. Arch. Biochem., **33**:259–62, 1951.
114. BERGDOLL, M. S. Unpublished data.

115. BERGDOLL, M. S., LAVIN, B., SURGALLA, M. J., and DACK, G. M. Science, **116**:633–34, 1952.
116. ELFORD, W. J. Proc. Roy. Soc. London, B, **112**:384, 1933.
117. LOWRY, O. H., ROSEBROUGH, N. J., FARR, A. L., and RANDALL, R. J. J. Biol. Chem., **193**:265, 1951.
118. JORDAN, EDWIN O., DACK, G. M., and WOOLPERT, ORAM. J. Prevent. Med., **5**:383–86, 1931.
119. MILLAR, E. L. M., and POWNALL, MARGARET. Brit. M. J., **2**:551–58, 1950.
120. GREENE, ROBERT A. J. Am. Osteopath. A., May, 1951.
121. NEVOT, A., BREVOT, G., PANTALEON, J., and ROSSET, R. Bull. Acad. vet., France, No. 3, March, 1951.
122. SURGALLA, M. J., and DACK, G. M. Food Technol., **7**:307–8, 1953.
123. SURGALLA, M. J., BERGDOLL, M. S., and DACK, G. M. J. Immunol., **72**:398–403, 1954.
124. SURGALLA, M. J. Unpublished data.
125. SURGALLA, M. J., BERGDOLL, M. S., and DACK, G. M. J. Immunol., **69**:357–65, 1952.
126. BAYLISS, MILWARD. J. Exper. Med., **72**:669–84, 1940.
127. BORISON, H. L., and WANG, S. C. Pharmacol. Rev., **5**:193, 1953.
128. RICHMOND, J. J., REED, C. I., SHAUGHNESSY, H. J., and MICHAEL, V. J. Bact., **44**:201, 1942.
129. ANDERSON, K. Brit. J. Exper. Path. & Bact., **34**:548, 1953.
130. SUGIYAMA, H. Unpublished data.
131. HOLTMAN, D. F., and PETERSON, W. A., JR. J. Bact., **64**:890, 1952.
132. SUGIYAMA, H., and DACK, G. M. J. Infect. Dis., **96**:286–94, 1955.

VI Salmonella

Perhaps no field is more confused than the one concerned with the role of the *Salmonella* organisms in food poisoning. *Salmonella*, a generic name applied to a group of bacteria which was formerly called "paratyphoid bacteria," was derived from D. E. Salmon, who, with Theobald Smith (1), first described a member of the group. There are numerous reasons why members of *Salmonella* are suspected in outbreaks of food poisoning. They have been known to be associated with it for many years when other types of bacteria were unrecognized, and bacteriologists automatically suspected members of the *Salmonella* group if *Clostridium botulinum* could not be implicated. Theories and conclusions have been advanced (as discussed later) which have falsely held that heat-stable products of *Salmonella* when ingested by man gave rise to symptoms of food poisoning. Therefore, it was not always considered necessary to recover the organism in culture. Some organisms have been isolated and called *Salmonella* but subsequently, upon thorough study, were found to be slow lactose fermenters belonging to the coliform group. Also, a positive diagnosis of *Salmonella* food poisoning might be incorrectly based upon a low titer of *Salmonella* agglutinins in the serum of patients. Thus many outbreaks have been reported as caused by *Salmonella* in which these microörganisms have had no part. The *Salmonella* group of bacteria is composed of many serotypes, with new ones still being described.

If *Salmonella* is ingested in large numbers by man, one or more of the following symptoms may follow: nausea, vomiting, abdominal cramping, and diarrhea; frequently fever and leukocytosis are also present.

DEFINITION

Salmonella are defined by Kauffmann (2) as follows: "The *Salmonella* group consists of serologically related, Gram-negative, aerobic, non-sporing rods, corresponding to *Salmonella typhi* in staining

159

properties and morphology, showing with certain exceptions, a motile, peritrichous phase in which they normally occur. They do not ferment adonitol, lactose, and sucrose, nor liquefy gelatin, nor produce indole, nor decompose urea, nor form acetylmethyl-carbinol. They regularly attack glucose with, but occasionally without gas production. They do not ferment salicin promptly, but in some cases delayed fermentation occurs." In addition, all members may be recognized by their antigenic structure. All types are pathogenic for man, animals, or both. Subsequently, in the definition, if strains do not fit the pattern with regard to fermentation of lactose or sucrose, liquefaction of gelatin, or production of indole, they are considered to belong to the *Salmonella* group if they contain O and H antigens typical of the group. The types of *Salmonella* which produce disease resembling typhoid fever in man are not considered here, since their epidemiology is identical to that of typhoid fever.

From 1923 to 1944 (3) 43 species, comprising 1,490 strains of *Salmonella*, have been isolated from cases or outbreaks of food poisoning in England and Wales. Of these strains, 56 were not identified for species. The commonest species arranged in order of prevalence are given in the accompanying table.

	No. Outbreaks		No. Outbreaks
S. typhimurium	665	S. montevideo	37
S. enteritidis	171	S. cholerae-suis	22
S. newport	159	S. bovis-morbificans	22
S. thompson	136	S. dublin	19
S. oranienburg	76	S. meleagridis	19

All *Salmonella* cultures ferment dextrose, usually with gas production, but not lactose or saccharose. *Salmonella typhimurium, S. enteritidis,* and *S. panama* ferment arabinose and trehalose with acid and gas, whereas *S. cholerae-suis* does not ferment these substances and is the only one of the four which fails to produce hydrogen sulphide. All four produce acid in tartrate medium (4), a fact which characterizes strains of animal origin.

The differentiation of a particular *Salmonella* is done by the agglutination test. This serological identification is made by antigenic analysis of somatic (O) and flagellar (H) antigens. By this test an antigenic formula has been given each of more than 150 species of *Salmonella*. In the formulas for antigenic structure in the

Kauffmann (5) and White (6) schema, the Roman numerals refer to the somatic (O) (cell body) antigen which divides the *Salmonella* strains into groups. The small letters and numbers refer to the flagellar (H) antigens. For example, *S. typhimurium* or *aertrycke* has the formula [I], IV, [V], XII: i:1, 2, 3, and *S. enteritidis* has [I], IX, XII : g, m:—. An International *Salmonella* Center has been established at the State Serum Institute, Copenhagen, which is financed by the Commonwealth Fund (7). This center supplies gratis to national *Salmonella* centers in the various countries some of the sera and cultures necessary for serological diagnosis and is prepared to examine doubtful cultures. In the United States, a National *Salmonella* Center is located at the Communicable Disease Center Laboratories of the United States Public Health Service, at Lawson, Georgia, under the direction of Dr. P. R. Edwards, who is also a member of the international committee. For a complete discussion of the serological identification test, the reader is referred to Kauffmann's book (5) or Circular No. 54, Kentucky Agricultural Experiment Station (8).

The problem of how fixed the antigenic components are, whether they may change and under what circumstances, is now under investigation in several laboratories. Perhaps the large number of types may be reduced, or simplified groupings made when more basic knowledge is discovered. The H antigens of *Salmonella* can be markedly changed by cultivating the organisms in serum containing agglutinins for the flagellar components (5). Edwards and Moran (9) reported the occurrence in nature of H antigens apparently identical with those obtained by cultivation of *Salmonella* in agglutinating serum. Subsequently, Bruner and Edwards (10) were successful in inducing changes in the O antigens of *Salmonella* by following a method in which absorbed O antisera were used in high concentration. Thus *S. anatum* was changed to a form indistinguishable from *S. newington,* and *S. meleagridis* to a form indistinguishable from *S. cambridge.*

HISTORICAL

The first outbreak of *Salmonella* described occurred in the village of Frankenhausen in Saxony, Germany, in 1888. As related by Gärtner (11), 57 persons became ill suddenly with symptoms of acute gastroenteritis. One young man who had consumed 800 gm. of raw meat died in about 35 hours. From the organs of this fatal case, Gärtner isolated a microörganism he named *Bacillus enteritidis*. He also isolated the same organism from the meat of the diseased cow which was responsible for the outbreak.

Another interesting case was described by Van Ermengem (12) in which several men ate sausages alleged to be responsible for the illness. A sanitary inspector of meat in a village of Belgium, who was reported to be a very famous veterinarian (M. L.), examined the incriminated sausages. Reassured by their excellent appearance, good odor, and color, he did not hesitate to declare them fit for consumption and volunteered to eat some to prove his absolute conviction of their harmlessness. M. D. K., the director of the slaughterhouse, and three workers also partook of the sausages. M. L. ate 3 slices at 11:00 A.M. on Saturday, October 26, 1895. After 10–12 hours he developed severe diarrhea and accompanying weakness, which continued and increased in severity. On Monday, when he called his physician, he had continuous diarrhea, violent colic, epigastric distress, pulse of 110, and temperature of 102° F. On Tuesday, the diarrhea persisted, with a foul-smelling yellowish discharge. The patient was restless and had precordial pain. The abdomen was not bloated; the urine was dark and contained a large quantity of albumin. There was manifest mydriasis, and the pupils reacted to light and to accommodation. On Tuesday the pulse was 100 and the temperature 101°5 F. On Wednesday morning the patient was delirious, prostrated, and had a temperature of 95°5 F. The stools were involuntary; the spleen and liver were enlarged. On Thursday the temperature was 97°9 F., and there was marked precordial pain. Thereafter the patient's condition became progressively worse, and he died at 6:00 A.M. Friday morning—or 6 days after eating the sausage. M. D. K. ate 3 or 4 slices of the sausage at approximately the same time. He said the meat had no abnormal taste but was strongly salted and spiced and seemed to have a metallic aftertaste, although this was not detected by M. L. On Sunday morning M. D. K. had diarrhea, with 5–6 stools, i.e., 20–24 hours had elapsed between the eating of the sausage and the onset of symptoms. At this time there was no colic, but the patient had a general feeling of illness. Diarrhea continued in the afternoon, with stools about every half-hour, and his appetite was poor. The next morning (Monday) stools were less frequent; the abdomen was tender, headache and lumbar pain were present, the pupils were dilated, and vision was blurred. On Tuesday urine was abundant, turbid, and brownish, verging on red. The stools were yellowish and fetid. Vision had returned to normal. Thereafter symptoms gradually abated, and recovery followed in a week. The accounts of the 3 workers were sketchy and incomplete. One man who had eaten 2 slices of sausage became ill in 28 hours, with fever, headache, general lassitude, frequent diarrhea, thirst, etc. The second who had tasted the sausage experienced nothing more than some abdominal discomfort, for which he took a laxative. The third who had eaten 1 slice from 3 different sausages given to him by M. L. had only a slight headache.

A necropsy was performed on M. L. and a diagnosis was made of acute gastroenteritis, probably infectious, with congestion and degeneration of the liver, acute parenchymatous nephritis, and pulmonary hyperemia. Typical *S. enteritidis* was isolated from the liver, spleen, lung, kidney, muscle (not as many colonies), portal blood (few), and the contents of the ileum. A mixture of liver and kidney from M. L. was injected subcutaneously, intraperitoneally, and by stomach tube into guinea pigs, rabbits, mice, rats, and dogs. All animals, except 2 dogs, died in a short time. Upon immediate examination after death, *S. enteriditis* was recovered from the animals' livers, kidneys, and other tissues. It is obvious, therefore, that M. L. had a septicemic infection, with the strain occurring naturally in animals. *Salmonella enteritidis* was isolated from the sausages; microscopic and chemical tests were negative for other agents or chemical poisons.

The outbreak described by Van Ermengem illustrates many important facts. In the first place, not all individuals react similarly, and the severity of symptoms is not proportional to the quantity of meat eaten. In the case of M. L., both the gastrointestinal and the septic types of disease were produced, whereas, in the other 4 individuals, only the gastrointestinal symptoms were manifested, and these were extremely mild in 3. Second, 12–24 or more hours elapsed from the time of eating the contaminated food to the first appearance of symptoms. This time interval provides an opportunity for *S. enteritidis* to multiply in the body and to invade the tissues.

PREVALENCE

The number of *Salmonella* outbreaks reported to the Public Health Service in the United States for the years 1951, 1952, and 1953 are given in the accompanying table (13–15). In these 67

Year	No. Out-breaks	Cases
1951............	15	850
1952............	31	1,335
1953............	21	533

outbreaks, 19 *Salmonella* types were identified; *S. typhimurium* accounted for 18. Nineteen of these outbreaks were attributed to chicken or turkey. Other foods involved were eggnog, egg yolk, baked Alaska, baked ham, spaghetti, chopped liver, homemade ice cream made from duck eggs, and cream filling from chocolate éclairs.

Felsenfeld, Young, and Yoshimura (16) studied 286 *Salmonella* strains isolated at the Cook County Hospital in Chicago, Illinois, between April 1, 1948, and November 25, 1950. Thirty-five types of *Salmonella* were found. The most frequently encountered were (in decreasing order), *S. typhimurium, S. typhosa, S. montevideo, S. oranienburg, S. newport, S. anatum, S. enteritidis,* and *S. paratyphi* B.

In England and Wales for the years 1949 through 1953 (17) 1,590 outbreaks[1] and family outbreaks[2] of food poisoning were reported. Of this number, 485 were caused by *Salmonella. S. typhimurium* accounted for 371, and other types of *Salmonella* for 114. Of the *S. typhimurium* outbreaks, 110 were due to contaminated processed meat, including gravy and stock, and 110 to contaminated duck eggs. Sweetmeats such as trifles, ice cream, cream cakes, custard, etc., were the vehicle of infection in 55 outbreaks. Thus these three classes of foods accounted for 74 per cent of the *S. typhimurium* outbreaks. Of the 114 outbreaks of other *Salmonella,* 60 were due to contaminated processed and made-up meat, including gravy and stock; 18 to contaminated sweetmeats; and 10 to duck

1. An "outbreak" refers to 2 or more related cases in persons in different families.

2. A "family outbreak" refers to 2 or more related cases in members of the same family.

eggs. Fish, milk, cheese, vegetables, and fruits accounted for a smaller number.

INCUBATION PERIOD

One of the most characteristic features of *Salmonella* gastrointestinal infections is the time required for symptoms to develop after the ingestion of the organism. This point is not stated clearly in most textbooks, because, in reports published before staphylococcus food

TABLE 12

CHARACTERISTICS OF *Salmonella* GASTROINTESTINAL INFECTIONS

Out-break	No. Cases	Causative Organism	Food	Onset of Symptoms (Hours)	Deaths
1 (18)....	18	*S. enteritidis*	Bread pudding	8–20	None
2 (19)....	135	*S. enteritidis* (?)	Milk contaminated with rat virus	12–48 (Peak 24–30)	None
3 (20)....	150	*S. cholerae-suis*	Milk	8–36	None
4 (21)....	65	*S. typhimurium*	Cheese	21–42	1
5 (22)....	31	*S. enteritidis*	Mutton	15–72	2
6 (23)....	52	*S. typhimurium*	Rice pudding made with infected duck eggs	7 and longer	1
7 (3).....	20	*S. oranienburg*	Scrambled eggs from dried eggs	12–40	None
8 (24)....	9	*S. berta*	Pork sausage	5–48	None
9 (25)....	1	*S. senegal*	Aspirated culture into mouth while pipetting	20	None
10 (26)....	1	*S. saint-paul*	Accidentally sucked suspension into mouth through un-plugged pipette	48	None
11 (13)....	41	*S. newport*	Sliced turkey, sliced tongue, potato salad	3–72	None

poisoning was generally recognized, food-poisoning outbreaks in which the incubation period was 2–3 hours were often ascribed to *Salmonella*. Present knowledge makes it possible to state that such outbreaks were, in all probability, due to staphylococci. Also characteristic is the variability in the time at which symptoms appear. These result from infection rather than from intoxication by preformed toxins; hence the incubation period varies with the time required for the multiplication and invasion by the organism in individuals having differing degrees of resistance.

In Table 12 a list of some carefully studied *Salmonella* outbreaks illustrates the length of the incubation period. In all instances the organsims were isolated from the patients and in some cases from the food as well. From these 523 cases, it can be seen that a period of at least 3 hours elapses before symptoms develop in the most susceptible individuals, 12–24 hours elapse in the majority of cases, and 24–30 hours or longer may elapse in a few cases. Finally, the fatalities are not high; out of the 523 cases, only 4 died.

SYMPTOMS

The symptoms of *Salmonella* gastrointestinal infection are characterized by nausea, vomiting, abdominal pain, and diarrhea. The onset often is sudden. The attack may begin with headache and chills. The abdominal pain, often the first symptom, may be griping and severe, accompanied with persistent, foul-smelling diarrhea. Later in the attack the stools may be watery and sometimes greenish in color. Prostration, muscular weakness, faintness, and thirst are marked. There are almost always a rise in temperature, various nervous manifestations of restlessness, muscular twitching, and drowsiness. Oliguria may be present, and herpes frequently follows.

The severity of the disease differs in various outbreaks and among individuals in the same outbreak. Dosage or number of organisms ingested is an important factor, since, in some experimental work as well, persons who have had a small dosage may escape without symptoms. All *Salmonella* organisms causing gastrointestinal upsets in man, however, seem to cause identical symptoms and to pursue the same course, regardless of the species involved. In a small percentage of cases the organisms may invade the tissues and cause death.

EPIDEMIOLOGY: *Salmonella* FOOD POISONING AN
   INFECTION? (27, 28)

Some years ago, when the *Salmonella* group was the principal one considered by bacteriologists in food outbreaks, actual search for the living organisms in incriminated foods often ended negatively. Therefore, investigators became interested in whether or not thermostable toxins or toxic products which would account for the outbreaks were produced. Savage and White (29, 30) found that a substance is produced by the bacteria which is definitely toxic to laboratory animals if injected intravenously or intraperitoneally. Other investigators (31, 32, 33) corroborated this work. Several (34, 35, 36) found that boiled *Salmonella* cultures, when fed to mice, caused death in a large proportion but might or might not be the cause of death when fed to other animals (37). G. Elkeles (38) has reviewed the literature on this subject.

In the reports dealing with the feeding of heat-killed *Salmonella* cultures to animals, the majority of positive results has been obtained with mice. Because the mouse reacts in this way, however, is no reason to assume that other species, including man, react similarly. As a matter of fact, the experimental evidence demonstrates that susceptibility in the mouse, as tested by the oral route, differs from that of other animals. For example, Bahr and Dyssegaard (32) fed rhesus monkeys up to 950 ml. (1 qt.) of heat-killed cultures over a period of about 4 days. The initial feeding, usually 250 ml., was followed by 2 other feedings of 350 ml. during the course of the next 3 days. No symptoms were observed, but appreciable agglutinins were demonstrated in the blood serum of the monkeys. In experiments carried out in our laboratory, heat-killed cultures of *S. typhimurium* fed to 4 rhesus monkeys failed (with 1 possible exception) to produce gastrointestinal symptoms characteristic of paratyphoid intoxication. On the other hand, living cultures of *S. typhimurium* and *S. enteritidis* fed to 11 rhesus monkeys caused watery diarrhea, general malaise, and in some cases loss of appetite (39). Recovery was prompt and apparently complete; the specific bacillus was not found in the blood stream. Monkeys fed with equivalent heat-killed portions of the same suspension showed no symptoms. Again, living cells of *Proteus* and *Escherichia coli* failed to produce any noticeable effect.

The crucial test as to whether or not heat-stable products of the food-poisoning types of *Salmonella* may cause illness in man rests upon feeding such material to humans. This has been done with negative results (33). Heat-killed, dextrose broth, beef heart cultures, and filtrates of 5 strains of *S. typhimurium* and 4 strains of *S. enteritidis*, when fed in amounts of 20–340 ml. (0.66–11 oz.) to 24 adults on an empty stomach, failed to produce any symptoms, although the same materials produced symptoms and death when injected intravenously into rabbits in 0.5–2-ml. amounts. No agglutinins for homologous strains were present in the serums of these subjects 10 days after feeding. One objection which may be raised to these experiments is that freshly isolated strains of *Salmonella* were not used. The answer may be found in the work of Verder and Sutton (40), who demonstrated that a living culture of *S. enteritidis* which had been under cultivation on artificial medium for 2 years produced typical symptoms of food poisoning when eaten in custards by a man. Moreover, heated suspensions, as well as unheated filtrates of a culture isolated from the stools and grown in custard, were fed to 7 human volunteers, none of whom became ill. Similarly, heated and filtered cultures of the same *S. enteritidis* strain produced no symptoms of food poisoning in monkeys, whereas living organisms, when fed, made the animals ill. From this experiment it is evident that filtrates or heat-stable products of a freshly isolated culture after passage through man are harmless when fed to humans.

Epidemiological evidence appears to corroborate the experimental evidence that living organisms are essential in outbreaks of food-borne infection caused by *Salmonella*. Hammerschmidt (41) stated that, in the course of an epidemic, only those people who ate uncooked or semicooked meat became ill, whereas others who ate cooked meat did not become ill. He also observed that people who did not eat the incriminated food were made ill by contact with persons who were actually ill. The evidence at the present time is overwhelmingly in favor of the view that *Salmonella* food poisoning is actually an infection and that toxins or toxic substances play no role.

SOURCES OF *Salmonella*

Human cases and carriers.—Edwards and Bruner (42) studied 224 cultures (excluding *S. paratyphi* A and *S. paratyphi* B) isolated from the stools of patients with gastroenteritis. The 10 most numerous species in order of importance are given in the accompanying table. In all, 39 species were studied. One hundred and eighteen

	No. Strains*		No. Strains*
S. typhimurium	43	S. sandiego	11
S. newport	31	S. bareilly	9
S. paratyphi B var. java	30	S. montevideo	9
S. panama	14	S. enteritidis	8
S. oranienburg	13	S. anatum	7

* Seven strains of *S. give* were also examined.

cultures from the stools of carriers were observed, and these were scattered among 24 species. Twenty-five cultures comprising 7 species were isolated from the stools of patients with enteric fever.

In four other laboratories (43–46) it was found that the prevalence of *Salmonella* species was at variance with those reported for England and Wales. *Salmonella panama* varied from the fifth to the tenth most prevalent species, and in three of the four collections, *S. anatum* varied from the third to the tenth. In general, *S. typhimurium*, *S. montevideo*, *S. oranienburg*, and *S. newport* were the types most frequently encountered.

Boyer and Tissier (47) described 4 epidemics of salmonellosis involving persons who had eaten horse meat purchased from a particular butcher-shop. These outbreaks illustrate the role of the carrier in spreading *Salmonella*. The majority of the people involved had eaten the meat after it was ground. It was evident that the meat was not contaminated when it left the wholesaler; half of the horse carcass which furnished the meat was sold to another butcher, and no illness had resulted. The sanitary conditions of the butcher-shop involved in the outbreak were satisfactory; no rat or mouse harborage was detected. Subsequently, however, it was established that the butcher's wife was a *Salmonella* carrier. She had helped her husband in handling the meat, cleaning the knives, grinding the meat, and cleaning the meat-grinder. The butcher's wife was removed from the market, and no further cases developed.

Household pets: cats.—Bruner and Moran (48) studied 34 *Salmonella* strains representing 17 different types of *Salmonella* isolated from cats. Mackel, Galton, Gray, and Hardy (49) isolated *Salmonella* types from 11 (12.1 per cent) of 91 cats which they examined.

Dogs.—*Salmonella* are propagated in the intestinal tracts of all domestic animals; the dog is no exception. Wolff and his co-workers (50) collected rectal swabs from 100 dogs and recovered *Salmonella* from 18. The following types were identified: *S. manhattan*, *S. newport*, *S. minnesota*, *S. oranienburg*, *S. typhimurium*, *S. bredeney*, *S. worthington*, *S. give*, *S. cubana*, *S. cerro*, *S. kentucky*, *S. illinois*, and *S. meleagridis*. In addition, 2 types were isolated which were not named.

Stucker, Galton, Cowdery, and Hardy (51) studied the prevalence and distribution of *Salmonella* in greyhounds in Florida. *Salmonella anatum*, *S. derby*, *S. newington*, *S. poona*, and *S. montevideo* were isolated. There was a relationship between the number of positive specimens and the sanitation in the kennels. In clean kennels, 32 per cent of the fecal specimens examined were positive for *Salmonella;* in kennels graded fair, 42 per cent were positive, whereas in those rated poor, 55 per cent of the specimens were positive.

Mackel, Galton, Gray, and Hardy (49) examined fecal specimens from normal family dogs through community surveys, rabies-immunization clinics, and veterinary hospitals (using dogs brought in for immunization, bathing, boarding, and surgical conditions). Forty-one types of *Salmonella* were obtained from 244 (15 per cent) *Salmonella* cultures isolated from 1,626 normal dogs.

Poultry: chickens, turkeys, ducks, and geese.—Hinshaw, McNeil, and Taylor (52) studied 561 *Salmonella* strains from 353 avian outbreaks caused by 23 types, 21 of which have also been found in man. *Salmonella typhimurium* was recovered in 60 per cent of 291 outbreaks in turkeys and in 35 per cent of 43 outbreaks in chickens. *Salmonella bareilly* caused 42 per cent of the outbreaks in chickens but only 5 per cent of those in turkeys.

Edwards, Bruner, and Moran (53) reported the occurrence and distribution of 60 *Salmonella* types among 6,387 cultures isolated from fowls. Of this number, 1,956 cultures were from 1,603 outbreaks in chickens; 4,007 from 2,390 outbreaks in turkeys. *Salmonella paratyphi* A was not found in fowls, but *S. paratyphi* B occurred in chickens and turkeys. Ninety-nine and one-half per cent of all *Salmonella* types isolated from fowls were found to belong to groups B, C, D, and E or were *S. worthington* or *S. minnesota.*

Corpron, Bivins, and Stafseth (54) demonstrated that mature bronze hen turkeys could be infected with *S. pullorum* both by feeding and by intravenous injection. After a period of 221 days some of the turkeys were found to be carriers of *S. pullorum.*

Gaumont (55) studied salmonellosis in fowls in northern France. In an examination of 245 birds or portions of birds originating from industry, farmers, and families of the northern and channel regions, 41 strains of *Salmonella* were isolated: 23 *S. gallinarum,* 13 *S. pullorum,* and 5 of other types.

Smith and Buxton (56) examined healthy adult domestic animals in England and Wales. They found *Salmonella* in 16 out of 650 turkeys, 2 out of 100 geese, 6 out of 500 ducks, and 5 out of 750 chickens.

Hemmes (57) isolated *S. bareilly* in the Netherlands. He reported that 9 patients had been infected by contact with chickens whose stools contained *S. bareilly*.

Edwards, Bruner, and Moran (53) found that tartrate-negative strains of *S. paratyphi* B, when fed to baby chicks, will produce a fatal septicemia. Milner and Shaffer (58) were able to infect young chicks with small numbers of organisms of many types of *Salmonella* by the oral route. Despite the benign course of the infection, they were able to find the organisms in the stools after a period of many days.

Hussemann and Wallace (59) injected chickens intravenously with *S. typhimurium* or *S. pullorum*. The chickens were bled 1 hour later to test for organisms in the circulating blood, then were slaughtered and broiled. These investigators found that the currently accepted methods of broiling or roasting markedly reduced the number of *Salmonella* present in chicken muscle or liver but never destroyed the entire inoculum. Two hundred and eighty samples of cooked fowl from public eating establishments were collected, and in no case were *Salmonella* found. Their negative tests with chickens from public eating establishments would indicate that their experimental tests with chickens intravenously injected with *Salmonella* were perhaps too severe to approximate naturally occurring *Salmonella* contamination of poultry meat.

Poultry products: fresh eggs.—Watt (60) made an excellent study of an outbreak of salmonellosis which he traced to shell eggs. *Salmonella montevideo* was isolated from 2 cases of shell eggs obtained from a merchant vessel. Twenty-eight individuals of a crew of 70 were affected after the consumption of contaminated egg salad. An attempt was made to trace the eggs to the farm, but this work had not been completed at the time of the report. Outbreaks of salmonellosis from duck eggs are well recognized, as Scott (61) pointed out.

Gernez-Rieux *et al.* (62) reported an outbreak due to *S. pullorum* in which 9 members of a healthy family ate their evening meal, consisting of vegetable bouillon, potatoes, and fried hen's eggs. The following morning 3 members of the family were ill with vomiting, abdominal cramps, profuse diarrhea, and fever. The symptoms lasted 48 hours, after which recovery was rapid. One of these strains, when fed to human volunteers by McCullough and Eisele (63) in dosages of 1,880,000, 13,900,000, and 110,000,000 organisms, caused no effect among 6 volunteers given each level; at a dosage of 1,280,000,000, 3 out of 6 men became ill. When the 6 men were fed 3,900,000,000 of this strain, 2 became ill. As discussed previously, these men had received yearly booster injections of typhoid vaccine, and, since the somatic antigen of *S. typhi* and *S. pullorum* is the same, some immunity to infection with *S. pullorum* may have been present.

Crowe (64) described an outbreak in which 23 out of 27 persons at risk developed salmonellosis. Apparently, a raw hen's egg infected with *S. typhimurium* was used in extending a butter ration. The process involved bringing a suspension of corn flour and milk to a boil, adding a quantity of butter and a raw egg, and whipping the ingredients together. The cook insisted that a hen's and not a duck's egg was used.

Mitchell, Garlock, and Broh-Kahn (65) reported an outbreak of gastroenteritis involving a known total of 423 persons, 172 of whom required hospitalization. *Salmonella pullorum* was isolated from 11.7 per cent of the hospitalized patients, and this organism was thought to have been the probable cause of the infections and to have been introduced into the rice pudding by infected eggs. The pudding was made with rice which had been boiled for 30 minutes. Raisins were cooked simultaneously. During these operations, chicken eggs were broken and the contents combined with canned milk and other ingredients. The rice was drained while still in the steam boiler and the raisins and egg mixture added without further heating, since the cooks thought that the rice contained enough heat to set the mixed pudding.

Carter, Powell, and Borts (66) examined 186 samples of eggs representing 247 dozen, or 2,964 eggs, taken from 56 cases (30 dozen per case). Positive cultures were found in 6 samples. *Salmonella paratyphi* B was recovered from 1 sample and *S. pullorum* from the remaining 5. Bernstein (67) examined the contents of 3,648 eggs from various sources and found no *Salmonella*.

Dried eggs.—During World War II, dried eggs were shipped in large quantities to Europe. Of 7,584 samples (3) from the United States, Canada, and Argentina, 754, or 9.9 per cent, were found to contain *Salmonella*. Thirty-three species were identified. In order of importance, the most common are listed.

	No. Isolated		No. Isolated
S. oranienburg	245	S. anatum	30
S. montevideo	139	S. typhimurium	30
S. meleagridis	117	S. newport	24
S. tennessee	90	S. senftenberg	8
S. bareilly	82	S. london	6

Twenty-two of the 33 species had not, as far as could be determined from published accounts, been encountered before 1941 in cases of infection in Great Britain. In 1943 there was an increase in cases out of proportion to what might have been anticipated that was attributed to *Salmonella*, and this occurred again in 1944. In a study of 428 outbreaks of food poisoning between 1923 and 1939, 14 species of *Salmonella* were identified as responsible for food-poisoning outbreaks, with not more than 9 species isolated in any one year. During the latter part of 1942, 1943, and 1944, outbreaks of food poisoning occurred which were due partly to the old *Salmonella* species and partly to 24 new species. Of the new types isolated, the predominant 6 headed the list of the dried-egg strains. From these facts the British concluded that dried eggs were probably responsible for a good proportion of the greatly increased number of outbreaks of food poisoning (67) during the years 1943 and 1944.

Gibbons and Moore (68) studied Canadian egg powder and isolated *Salmonella* organisms from 28 of 380 samples. *Salmonella* counts made on 21 samples showed that 13 contained less than 1 organism per gram, 7 between 1 and 10, and 1, 54 per gram.

Solowey, McFarlane, Spaulding, and Chemerda (69) isolated *Salmonella* from 35 per cent of 5,198 samples of spray-dried whole-egg powder obtained from 100 dehydration plants between September, 1943, and January, 1945. The incidence varied from 0 to 71 per cent for individual plants. Fifty-two *Salmonella* types were identified. *Salmonella pullorum, S. oranienburg, S. montevideo, S. tennessee,* and *S. anatum* totaled 73 per cent of the isolations.

Professor G. Olin (70), director of the State Bacteriological Laboratory in Stockholm, Sweden, reported studies made by Professor Sven Gard and Dr. Ernst Hammarstrom. During the latter part of

1945, all of 1946, and the first half of 1947, new *Salmonella* types for Sweden were diagnosed. These new types were *S. oranienburg, S. kentucky, S. tennessee, S. bareilly, S. niloese, S. senftenberg,* and *S. meleagridis.* Some previous species that had been isolated occasionally were found in increasing numbers, such as *S. panama, S. montevideo,* and *S. thompson.* Furthermore, on repeated stool examinations, combinations of *Salmonella—S. bareilly, S. oranienburg,* and *S. montevideo*—were isolated from 1 case; *S. oranienburg* and *S. tennessee* were isolated in combination in 2 patients; and *S. montevideo* and *S. worthington* both were found in 1 case. Again, other *Salmonella* were isolated from individual cases within the same family. Since many types of *Salmonella* were found in dried-egg powder and the new ones were those discovered in imported dried eggs, the source of the new types was explainable. An examination of 260 imported dried-egg powders from the United States revealed 72 unusual serotypes, with 28.1 per cent of the specimens containing *Salmonella.* Of 173 specimens from South America, 26.6 per cent contained *Salmonella;* and of 825 specimens from Denmark, 0.5 per cent contained *Salmonella.*

In 1952 (14) canned dried egg-yolk powder fed to infants was reported responsible for cases of salmonellosis. *Salmonella montevideo* was demonstrated in samples of certain code numbers of the egg product and in the stools of sick infants. Although the canned dried egg-yolk powder was heated before drying, the treatment was not sufficient to destroy all *Salmonella.* The author made a study of *S. montevideo* infections in 7 institutions where *Salmonella* were regularly typed. The work was concerned with children from birth to two years for 1950, 1951, and 1952. Illnesses in this age group caused by *S. montevideo* occurred during all 3 years, but the incidence was higher in the last quarter of 1952. Whether the increase was due to the contaminated egg product or to the publicity, causing more cases to be recognized, cannot be answered.

Effect of heat treatment of eggs on Salmonella.—Solowey and Calesnick (71) have shown that procedures like frying and boiling eggs in the shell, as well as scrambling, do not heat the eggs sufficiently to destroy *Salmonella.* Goresline, Hayes, Moser, Howe, and Drewniak (72) studied the pasteurization of liquid whole egg, under commercial condition, to eliminate *Salmonella.* They reported that milk-pasteurizing equipment may be used, with little or no change, for the pasteurization of liquid whole egg. Winter (73) found that pasteurization of whole eggs or yolks at 142° F. for 2 minutes and whites at 134° F. for 2 minutes will destroy more than 99 per cent of the bacteria and improve their storage quality without injuring the functional properties. Anellis, Lubas, and Rayman (74) determined the heat resistance of strains of *Salmonella* in liquid eggs sealed in thermal death time glass tubes for heating. The antigenic type and strain and the pH of the liquid egg in which the organisms were suspended were factors affecting the thermal resistance of the organisms. At least twofold more time at constant temperature was required for bacterial destruction at pH 5.5 than at 8.0. Osborne, Straka, and Lineweaver (75) tested the heat resistance of several strains of *Salmonella* in liquid whole egg, egg white, and egg yolk. A shorter thermal time in the pH region of 8.0–9.0 than in the region of pH 5.5–7.5 was found. All strains were more stable in liquid whole egg than in phosphate buffer or egg white. One strain of *S. senftenberg* was observed to have a several fold longer thermal death time than any other strain of *Salmonella* tested.

Ayres (76) developed a procedure for determining the amount of *Salmonella* contamination in dried-egg products. Weighed samples (0.1, 1.0, and 10 gm.) were handled aseptically and put into flasks containing 3, 9, and 90 ml. of Selenite-F enrichment broth; five flasks for each of the three different weights were used. The flasks were incubated at 37° C. for 16–20 hours, after which a loopful from each flask was streaked on Kauffmann's Brilliant Green Agar. The plates were incubated for 24 hours, and *Salmonella* colonies appeared as pinkish-white opalescent colonies surrounded by a bright-red area. If the colonies were typical for *Salmonella* in subsequent biochemical tests, then the number of positive plates for each dilution was compared with the corresponding number in probability tables.

Fermented egg albumen is difficult to process free from *Salmonella*, since heat interferes with its functional use. Clinger, Young, Prudent, and Winter (77) found that egg white pasteurized for 4 minutes at 57° C. produced undesirable angel-food cakes unless the standard beating procedure was modified. Ayres and Slosberg (78) observed that fermented egg albumen flash-pasteurized at 139° F.

contained no viable *Salmonella* but that recontamination occurred in holding vessels and drying, and also that hydrogen peroxide at levels of 0.1 and 0.2 per cent, followed by removal of the residual hydrogen peroxide with excess catalase, destroyed all organisms of the *Salmonella* group. It was their experience that storage of the dried fermented albumens at room temperature did not eliminate living *Salmonella*, although storage at 120°, 130°, and 135° F. for 20, 8, and 4 days, respectively, was successful in getting rid of enteric pathogens without affecting the beating rates.

Frozen egg whites have on occasion been associated with salmonellosis outbreaks. Baked Alaska, a dessert made with ice cream, cake, and beaten egg white and browned in a hot oven before serving, was incriminated in one outbreak. Approximately 60 per cent of 600 guests became ill the morning after an evening meal at which baked Alaska was served. *Salmonella montevideo* was found in a sample of the frozen egg whites but was not detected in rectal cultures taken during convalescence from 14 people who became ill. Since the symptoms and incubation period were consistent with *Salmonella* infection and no other common food item or causative agent was found, the outbreak was believed to have been caused by *S. montevideo*.

Swine.—Hormaeche and Salsamendi (79) studied *Salmonella* infections in children in Montevideo, Uruguay. In searching for sources of these infections, the mesenteric lymph glands of apparently normal hogs slaughtered for the market were examined. Forty-six lots of hogs, each consisting of 20 animals, revealed that 47.9 per cent yielded *Salmonella* organisms. Rubin, Scherago, and Weaver (80) cultured the mesenteric lymph glands from 40 lots of hogs of 25 animals each; 47.5 per cent of the lots contained *Salmonella*. Of 50 hogs studied individually, in which the mesenteric lymph nodes were cultured, 5 yielded *Salmonella*. The frequency of the types found by these workers is given in the accompanying table.

S. typhimurium	7	S. derby	2
S. cholerae-suis	4	S. new brunswick	2
(var. Kunzendorf)		S. bredeney	1
S. oregon	4	S. enteritidis	1
S. anatum	3	S. lexington	1
S. give	3	S. newington	1
S. bareilly	2	S. worthington	1

In these experiments (79, 80), enrichment methods of culture were used which are selective and would reflect small numbers of *Salmonella* present. It is doubtful whether the *Salmonella* recovered represented invasion of the lymph nodes, since no controls were made to eliminate surface fecal contamination which occurs normally in slaughtering operations. Only under aseptic measures, such as those used in abdominal surgery and before the bowel is cut, could bacteriological specimens of mesenteric lymph nodes be obtained. It may well be, therefore, that the *Salmonella* which were obtained reflected fecal contamination and not *Salmonella* which had invaded the mesenteric lymph nodes. From the public health standpoint there may be significant differences in the dosage or numbers of *Salmonella* contaminating meat. In the case of tissue invasion, the dosage may be greater than the natural fecal contamination from the carcasses of carrier animals.

Kraneveld, Erber, and Mansjoer (81) cultured the mesenteric lymph nodes of 150 normal pigs from six farms in the area of Bogor, West Java. *Salmonella* were isolated from 25 of these animals. Clarenburg, Vink, and Huisman (82) observed *Salmonella* in the mesenteric lymph nodes of 14 of 503 healthy pigs but none in the stools. Gaumont (83) examined the mesenteric lymph nodes of 147 pigs and recovered *Salmonella* in 6. Kämpe, Lilleengen, and Österling (84) examined 93 hogs slaughtered during the winter and spring. Feces, mesenteric lymph nodes, liver, bile, spleen, and kidneys were cultured for *Salmonella*, and none was found. The mesenteric lymph nodes were examined from 1,980 hogs slaughtered during the autumn and distributed into 202 groups. From 14 groups of hogs, 15 *Salmonella* strains were isolated. Smith and Buxton (56) isolated *Salmonella* from 4 fecal specimens from 600 healthy pigs. From these studies it is obvious that salmonellosis in swine is prevalent throughout many different countries.

Galton, Smith, McElrath, and Hardy (85) discovered *Salmonella* in 25 per cent of 100 fecal specimens of hogs in the abattoir, whereas, on the farm, only 7 per cent of 374 specimens were positive. These findings were attributed to the swine's becoming infected during transportation or in the holding lots. Although no clinical evidence was presented, Galton *et al.* make the statement: "Apparently, many may be killed during the incubation stage of subclinical or

clinical salmonellosis." Galton, Lowery, and Hardy (86) made 217
examinations of fresh sausage for *Salmonella*. In fresh pork sausage
marketed by local Florida abattoirs, 57.5 per cent of 40 samples
were positive. From 79 samples of fresh sausage from national distributors, only 7.5 per cent were positive. Twenty-two samples of
smoked sausage from local abattoirs were examined for *Salmonella*;
40.9 per cent were positive. In 49 samples of smoked sausage from
national distributors, no *Salmonella* was found. One hundred and
twenty-two cultures of 19 types of *Salmonella* were recovered from
sausage, 44 *S. derby*, 39 *S. anatum*, 6 *S. bredeney*, 5 *S. newport*,
and the 15 types remaining represented 4 or less serotypes each. The
authors suggest that there may be a difference in the *Salmonella* content between fresh products and those stored for varying lengths of
time or that there may be true regional variations in the incidence
of infection in hogs. No evidence was presented to explain the lower
incidence of *Salmonella* in the sausage of national distributors. They
also reported that in Florida, of the 12 most common types of
Salmonella found in man, 9 were among the 12 most common
types in swine.

Galton *et al.* (86) examined rectal swabs from 1,196 cattle from
seven dairies in Florida for *Salmonella*. All 596 cultures taken from
five herds were negative; 2 positive cultures—*S. give* and *S. bareilly*
—were obtained from one herd of 50 cows. In a large herd of 550
animals, including calves, heifers, and cows, 14 were positive for
Salmonella. The types isolated were *S. give*, *S. anatum*, and *S. kentucky*. *Salmonella* was found in 17 of 147 fecal specimens of both
hogs and cattle taken immediately after slaughter in abattoirs in
Florida.

Cattle.—Smith and Buxton (56) found *S. dublin* in 3 of 750 fecal
specimens from cattle. Lilleengen and Mickow (87) failed to find
Salmonella in mesenteric lymph glands of 106 cattle and 102 young
calves. Bruner and Moran (48), in an analysis of 16 years' experience typing *Salmonella* cultures, studied cultures from 69 outbreaks
in cattle, compared to 1,056 for swine and 4,658 for fowl. From
their work it is apparent that salmonellosis in cattle is uncommon as
compared to that in fowl and swine.

Cherry, Scherago, and Weaver (88) examined various types of
meat products from retail markets by a cultural enrichment method

for isolating *Salmonella* species. Of 250 samples examined, 13, or 5.2 per cent, contained *Salmonella*, with the incidence in pork products greater than in beef. Again, this study may reflect the small amount of fecal contamination incident to slaughtering. With our knowledge of *Salmonella* species in nature increasing, it does not now appear that the utopia of *Salmonella*-free domestic animals will be reached. The low incidence of *Salmonella* food-poisoning outbreaks in man would indicate that our methods of handling and cooking meats are satisfactory.

Meat poisoning, despite its obscure meaning to German workers, generally refers to *Salmonella* infection of the food-poisoning type, although food poisoning by bacteria other than *Salmonella* may be caused by contaminated meat. Foods other than meats, however, have been implicated in many outbreaks of *Salmonella* infection (18–23). Milk and cheese from a diseased cow may become contaminated by the cow or upon subsequent handling by the milk processors.

Rodents.—In nature, rats and mice may be a reservoir of *Salmonella*. The subject of natural infections in rodents is reviewed by Bartram, Welch, and Ostrolenk (89), who found that fatal infections often follow the feeding of rats with massive doses of *S. enteritidis*. On the other hand, more uniform and lasting infections are obtained with one small dose. In some instances, upon the first day and lasting as long as 34 days, positive fecal specimens were obtained from 15 out of 24 rats fed 100 organisms. That rats may be carriers was suggested by the intermittent excretion of the infecting organism for at least 7 weeks. Continued high agglutinin titers were obtained for 4 months after infection. Transmission of the infection from an infected rat to cage mates was demonstrated; recovery of the infective organism from the composite feces and from individual rats lasted as long as the fortieth day after contact with an infected animal. Examination of feces from 800 white laboratory rats and agglutination tests on the blood of 26 showed the absence of *Salmonella* infection. These workers (90) in a later report noted that excreta of rats infected with *S. enteritidis* held at room temperature may contain living organisms for at last 148 days, and also that infection of rats and mice with very few organisms is possible when they are fed a virulent strain of *S. enteritidis* by stomach tube. Bartram *et al.*

were able to transfer the infection from an infected animal to cage mates through seven colonies of rats and three of mice.

A study of the excreta of rats and mice collected in areas throughout the United States indicates that only a small percentage (1.2 per cent) excrete food-poisoning organisms of the *Salmonella* type. This small percentage may be attributed in part to the limitations of the laboratory methods employed by the authors, who streaked only plates of bismuth sulphite agar from tetrathionate enrichment cultures of feces. The incidence of infection in wild rats and mice is reported:

> The results of examining some 420 specimens of rat and mice pellets, from which only five strains of *Salmonella* of the food poisoning type were isolated, collected throughout the country, however, might explain the dearth of food poisoning outbreaks proved to be the result of infected rodents. It is true that much higher incidences of food poisoning organisms have been reported in rats and mice, but invariably the investigators reporting such figures gathered their animals in a small area, or from a definite source, such as a packinghouse or bakery and in several instances the studies were carried out because of a recent outbreak. Under such conditions with the apparent ease of transmission of infection in rat colonies higher incidences of infection in a given area might be expected [90].

The role of rats in the spread of *Salmonella* infections of the food-poisoning type is summarized:

> Although a much larger series of specimens of rodent excreta need to be examined from many more areas in the United States before a definite conclusion can be reached, our studies to date indicate that relatively few rodents are infected with food poisoning organisms of the *Salmonella* group. It would appear that this would explain, in part at least, the relatively few outbreaks of food poisoning in which rodents were proved to be vectors of the causative organisms. Nevertheless, since some few rats or mice may be infected with food poisoning organisms, they all must be considered potentially dangerous to health, and every effort should be made to eliminate them from establishments where human food is prepared or stored [90].

Salmonella organisms have been used in an attempt to exterminate rats. The incorrectness of such procedure is illustrated not only by the experimental work detailed (89, 90) but by outbreaks which have been directly traceable to this procedure. Spray (19) in 1926 reported an outbreak of 135 cases probably due to milk contaminated with rat "virus." The commercial rat virus was distributed around the kitchen, serving-room, and storerooms 16 days before the outbreak. A bag of the rat virus bait obtained from the serving-room was found to contain viable bacteria identical with strains isolated from patients. The virus lay on the floor, which was washed daily with a hand-wrung string mop. The kitchen assistant who mopped the floor performed other duties, such as washing dishes and preparing salads.

Insects.—The housefly (*Musca domestica*) was found responsible for spreading enteric diseases. During the Boer (91) and Spanish-American wars (92), thousands of cases of typhoid fever were traced to the contamination of food by flies. In an experimental study of the housefly as a vector of food-poisoning organisms in food establishments (93), it was found that the number of bacteria deposited is determined by the type of material upon which the flies feed. When *S. enteritidis* was experimentally inoculated on food, flies were found to infect other flies, food, water, and surfaces with which they came in contact. *Salmonella enteritidis* were found in maggots, pupae, and adult flies coming in sequence from contaminated fly eggs. The organism was found to survive in the fly for its life-duration, or approximately 4 weeks. In view of these experiments, it is obvious that flies can play an important role in the spread of food-borne infections and that foods should be protected.

Eskey, Prince, and Fuller (94) found that the 2 common rat fleas, *Xenopsylla cheopis* and *Nosopsyllus fasciatus,* may be infected with *S. enteritidis* when feeding upon infected mice and that the fleas may transmit the infection from one mouse to another by their bites. Feces of infected fleas were observed to contain large numbers of viable *S. enteritidis.* More than half of the fleas remained infected with *S. enteritidis* until death, the organisms causing a pathological condition in the alimentary canal.

Olson and Rueger (95), using three common species of household roaches as potential carriers, conducted a series of transmission experiments with *S. oranienburg.* Their survival was determined by an examination of the feces. The test strain was found to exist 10 days in the American roach, 12 in the German, and 20 in the oriental. In the latter, a post mortem examination showed that *S. oranienburg* survived 42 days after an infective feeding, although the insect had passed contaminated feces only during the first 20 days.

Nonanimal products.—Some outbreaks have been attributed to nonanimal products, such as dried foods made of cereal and dried yeast. In these instances the source of contamination is unknown. In England and Wales (17) for the year 1950, there were 134 outbreaks and family outbreaks in which the presumed causal agent was *S. typhimurium*. Of these outbreaks, 21 were from sweet dishes, 4 from vegetables, 2 from fruit, and 1 from sauce.

A strain of *S. enteritidis* was experimentally inoculated into cans of asparagus, spinach, string beans, tomato juice, peaches, shrimp, salmon, corn, and peas (96). Duplicate cans were incubated at 22° and 37° C. Growth occurred in asparagus, peas, corn, spinach, string beans, tomato juice, shrimp, and salmon incubated at 22° C., and in peas, corn, spinach, string beans, tomato juice, salmon, and shrimp at 37° C. *Salmonella enteritidis* appeared to grow better and last longer at 22° C. than at 37° C. In asparagus, string beans, tomato juice, and peaches, viable organisms were found at 22° C. after 30 and 60 days, whereas after 30 days at 37° C. no viable organisms could be detected except in the string beans. Obviously, *Salmonella* are not found in unopened canned foods, since the processing times and temperatures of canning preclude their survival. Therefore, *Salmonella* food poisoning from canned foods can occur only where the can has been opened and contaminated with the organism. Under natural circumstances, pure cultures of *Salmonella* would not contaminate foods, and the multiplication of these organisms in foods would be competitive with other naturally occurring contaminants.

HUMAN VOLUNTEERS FED *Salmonella*

McCullough and Eisele (63, 97, 98) fed human volunteers strains of *Salmonella* isolated from market samples of spray-dried whole-egg powder by Solowey and co-workers (69). They used six species—three strains each of *S. meleagridis* and *S. anatum;* one each of *S. newport, S. derby,* and *S. bareilly;* and four of *S. pullorum.* The number of organisms was given in increasing dosages until illnesses occurred. All strains caused illness in human volunteers, and the dosage was found to be different for strains of the same type. In the case of one strain of *S. anatum,* illnesses were caused when 587,000 organisms were fed, whereas, with another strain, 44,500,-000 organisms were needed. With *S. pullorum,* 1,000,000,000 or more cells were required. However, the authors noted that these strains contain the same somatic antigen as that represented in the periodic booster injections of typhoid vaccine given to the volunteers. Further work is necessary to determine whether typhoid vaccine offers protection against infection with *S. pullorum*.

In McCullough and Eisele's studies the time from the ingestion of the cultures to the onset of symptoms ranged from $3\frac{1}{2}$ hours to 7 days. In 433 individual feedings there were 73 illnesses; in 3 cases (4.1 per cent) the incubation period was less than 5 hours, and in 42 (57 per cent) the incubation period was 24 hours or less. Twenty-three of the subjects who became ill after the ingestion of either *S. meleagridis* or *S. anatum* were refed these organisms (99). Increased resistance was observed, although the degree of insusceptibility varied. Six of 7 subjects who developed prolonged carrier states in the initial experiments promptly ceased excreting organisms after refeeding. All the strains fed to human volunteers were injected intra-abdominally into mice to determine the ID_{50} (100). There was no relationship between the pathogenicity of these strains for human volunteers and the ID_{50} for mice.

Frequently, with small dosages the volunteer might not become ill and yet become a carrier. In small dosages the carrier state might not be detected for several days.

LABORATORY DIAGNOSIS OF *Salmonella* AS THE CAUSE OF
GASTROINTESTINAL UPSETS

The best diagnosis may be attained when *Salmonella* are found in both stools and suspected food. Unfortunately, this goal is not often attainable. According to Verder and Sutton (40), the smaller the number of organisms swallowed, the longer the incubation period. However, during the time of acute symptoms almost pure cultures of *Salmonella* may be recovered—a fact which indicates that *S. enteritidis* may supplant the normal fecal flora. Thereafter, the organisms rapidly disappear from the stools. Often outbreaks are not studied until acute symptoms have subsided, and the causative bacterium is not always present. Suspected foods may be ground with sterile sand in a sterile mortar and streaked on appropriate media, but the incriminated foods are frequently not available for testing.

There are several selective media for culturing *Salmonella*. In our experience, the *Salmonella-Shigella* (SS) medium, manufactured in dehydrated form by the Digestive Ferments Company, has been found excellent. *Escherichia coli* is inhibited on this medium, and the majority of strains of *Salmonella* can be detected. Small numbers of *Salmonella* and those strains which do not grow on SS medium may develop in enrichment cultures in tetrathionate broth or Selenite-F medium (101). Subinoculations may then be made into differential media.

The technical methods of identifying suspicious nonlactose fermenting colonies of bacteria occurring on plated media are sufficiently described in textbooks of bacteriology to warrant omission here. Since the final serological tests to determine antigenic structure require a number of strains and antisera which most laboratories do not possess, it is advisable to send cultures to a laboratory equipped for this work.

Savage and White (29), studying cases of food poisoning in which *Salmonella* were suspected but no living organisms could be found in the food, tested for the presence of specific toxic substances by the following three methods: (1) the production of gastrointestinal irritation in rabbits fed suspected food; (2) the demonstration of specific agglutinins in patients' sera; and (3) the injection of animals with extracts of the suspected food and the demonstration of specific agglutinins in their sera. The discussion which follows indicates that none of these methods is reliable.

The first method consisted of feeding suspected food to young rabbits, killing them in 9–12 hours, and examining their stomachs and duodenums. Post mortem examinations showed various degrees of hyperemia of the mucosa, with little correlation between severity of hyperemia and dosage, strain, etc. Dack, Harmon, and Jarra (37) repeated these experiments with negative results on 17 rabbits killed by suffocation.

Savage and White (29) stated that their second criterion was not reliable. The agglutination titers were all low (only 2 above 1:100) and in many cases were negative. Where there was definite agglutination, the titer varied considerably from day to day. They explain the lack of agglutinins in some patients by the rapid expulsion of antigen, owing to the diarrhea and vomiting, and in others by the ingestion of the toxic food after it was well cooked. These authors could demonstrate no agglutinins in laboratory animals which had been fed boiled cultures. Similarly, the experience of others has indicated that the agglutinin titer in the sera of individuals experiencing an attack of *Salmonella* infection of the food-poisoning type is frequently not high. Some 10 days after an attack, Rosenau and Weiss (18) tested the sera of 3 patients with the specific organism isolated from food. Agglutination was found to occur in a dilution of 1:100 of patient's serum but not in 1:500. Culley (22) tested sera from 29 patients 10 days after an attack. In 19 he found titers ranging from 1:25 to 1:500, and the remaining 10 sera from patients with mild attacks did not agglutinate the specific strain in a 1:25 dilution. Verder and Sutton (40) tested the serum, at the time of illness and again 10 days after recovery, of a volunteer who was made ill with *S. enteritidis.* At the onset of illness the specific organism was partially agglutinated in 1:20 and 1:40 dilutions and, 10 days later, in 1:80 and 1:160 dilutions. Moreover, monkeys which were fed living *Salmonella* cultures (41) and developed gastrointestinal symptoms characteristic of those occurring in outbreaks in man did not develop an appreciable agglutinin titer.

The third of Savage and White's criteria is not valid because the results can be interpreted differently. Owing to the prevalence of *Salmonella* infections in domestic animals and rodents, the tested animals may have a low titer of antibody due to previous slight infections. This titer may increase after the injection of a foreign antigen, for example, a suspected food, since the intravenous injection of any antigen increases the titer of all antibodies present in the serum (anamnestic phenomenon). No titer reported by Savage and White was higher than 1:200; the average titer was lower, and no control with bland protein was recorded.

As stated, it is necessary to demonstrate living *Salmonella* in specimens submitted for bacteriological examination in order to substantiate a diagnosis of *Salmonella* infection of the food-poisoning type.

CONTROL

The control of *Salmonella* in foods presents a difficult and serious problem to the food-processor. Since *Salmonella* are widespread in nature, they have appeared in dried foods of nonanimal origin. Often the first indication a processor may have of *Salmonella* is when a gastrointestinal illness follows the consumption of his product and the same *Salmonella* type is recovered from both patient and product. Where the food is not subjected to cooking before serving, it is recalled from the market. Food-processors dealing with products which do not require cooking should give thought to the potential *Salmonella* hazard involved.

Although large outbreaks of *Salmonella* infection are not common in the United States, there are no records of the number of cases that occur within the individual family. Dosage seems to be an important factor in the occurrence of infection. Perishable foods or foods serving as a medium for the growth of *Salmonella* contaminants should be kept under refrigeration to prevent an effective dosage of *Salmonella* from developing.

From the evidence available it appears that small numbers of *Salmonella* may find their way into the majority of kitchens, but, with the method of food handling practiced in the United States, few *Salmonella* cases result. There is ample experimental evidence, however, that where *Salmonella* are present as contaminants in food, their numbers will increase under favorable conditions of time and temperature. Undercooking may provide incubation time and temperature for multiplication of *Salmonella*. This is well illustrated in an outbreak reported to the Public Health Service by Dr. F. S. Leeder, Michigan Department of Health (102). Of 250 people who partook of a turkey dinner, 2 died and 161 became sufficiently ill to consult doctors. Turkey dressing was believed responsible when *S. typhimurium* was found in the stuffing and not in a specimen of the turkey meat. Dressing may be an excellent insulation material, and again, unless sufficient time and temperature in cooking are allowed, *Salmonella* in the center of the stuffing may not be destroyed and may, in fact, multiply.

Under interstate commerce, meat is inspected by federal agents. This means that animals suffering from *Salmonella* infections are eliminated. The United States federal meat-inspection act was approved June 30, 1906, for one year, extended on March 18, 1907, and amended in 1913, 1919, 1922, and 1930. The law provides for the inspection of meat or animal products which are shipped interstate or into foreign countries. Cattle, sheep, goats, swine, and, in a restricted way, horses are included.

The purpose of meat inspection is to prevent the sale of diseased or unhealthy meat and to see that clean and sanitary conditions are provided for the preparation and processing of foods composed entirely or partly of meat. The use of harmful dyes, preservatives, chemicals, or other deleterious substances is forbidden. False and misleading labels and statements are not permitted. The inspection services carried out by the Meat Inspection Branch of the Agricultural Research Service, which administers the law, are divided as follows: (1) sanitation; (2) ante mortem, or live-animal inspection; (3) post mortem, or slaughter inspection; (4) products inspection, or supervision of processing and manufacturing meat-food products; and (5) laboratory inspection.

In regard to sanitation, meat-storage places must be ratproof. On the slaughtering floors the equipment must be properly sterilized and free from contamination before being used on sound carcasses. A pure water supply and good drainage also must be provided. The ante mortem inspection eliminates the majority of sick animals. Under this examination, animals sick from *Salmonella* infections are detected and are not sold as food. An outbreak, such as that described by Gärtner (11), in which a sick cow was slaughtered and the meat salvaged and sold, could not have occurred if the animal had been properly inspected beforehand. The evidences of *Salmonella* infection are recognizable by the experienced meat inspector, and diseased animals that pass the ante mortem inspection are discovered and condemned at post mortem. The final inspection also serves to guard against contamination of the products during manufacture (curing, etc.) after slaughter. The scarcity of *Salmonella* outbreaks from meat products in this country is probably a true measure of the effectiveness of our methods of meat inspection. Further, our excellent federal meat-inspection procedures have served as an example to municipalities which have to deal with small abattoirs furnishing meat used locally.

Salmonella INVOLVED IN GASTROINTESTINAL INFECTIONS

Salmonella aertrycke is now referred to as *S. typhimurium* Castellani and Chalmers 1919, since Loeffler in 1890 isolated it from a mouse epizoötic. However, it is known under many names—such as *Bacterium psittacosis*, Nocard, 1893; *Bacillus kaensche* Breslau bacillus, von Kaensche, 1896; *B. aertrycke*, De Nobele, 1899, 1901;

B. pestiscaviae, Wherry, 1908; *B. paratyphosus* B mutton type, von Schütze, 1920; Group VII, von Hecht-Johansen, 1923; *S. aertrycke,* Ibrahim and Schütze, 1928, Warren and Scott, 1929–30, and Bruce White, 1929–30. In the German literature *Salmonella* has been called *Mäusetyphus-Bacillus* and *Bact. enteritidis* Breslau. The antigenic structure (5) is [I], IV, [V], XII:i:1, 2, 3.

Salmonella typhimurium has been found in more food-poisoning outbreaks than any other species of *Salmonella.* Its numerous names are sufficient evidence of the confusion existing from attempts of bacteriologists at classification. Epizoötics among rabbits and guinea pigs have been frequently traced to *S. typhimurium,* which has caused extensive outbreaks of dysentry and diarrheal disease among sheep and calves. Nocard believed *S. Typhimurium* was the cause of psittacosis since it was isolated from sick parrots, but it is now well recognized that psittacosis is caused by a filtrable virus.

Salmonella enteritidis Castellani and Chalmers, 1919, was isolated in 1888 by Gärtner in a meat-poisoning epidemic in Frankenhausen. Gärtner called it *B. enteritidis.* Another synonym is Typhus Gärtner Jena, Kauffmann, 1930, 1931. The antigenic structure (5) is [I], IX, XII . . . g, m . . . —. Three varieties have been distinguished based upon biochemical differences.

Salmonella enteritidis, found less frequently in food-poisoning outbreaks than *S. typhimurium,* produces the same symptoms clinically. It is the cause of epizoötics among many species of animals. Calves are susceptible to infection with this organism, and rats and mice are found naturally infected with either or both *S. enteritidis* and *S. typhimurium.*

Salmonella newport was first isolated from man in England (103). Since that time it has also been found in numerous animal species (42), including fowls, ruminants, swine, carnivores, and rodents. *Salmonella newport* has the antigenic formula VI, VIII:e, h:1, 2, 3. . . .

Salmonella oranienburg was first isolated from the feces of a healthy child in Germany. It has been found both in fowl and in man (104), and there is considerable evidence supporting its pathogenicity for man. It has the following antigenic formula: VI, VII: m, t:—.

Salmonella montevideo was first reported by Hormaeche and

Peluffo (105) in Uruguay from monkeys, swine, and children. It has a wide geographic distribution and has been found in fowl, swine, carnivores, and man (42). It has the antigenic formula VI, VII: g, m, s:—.

Salmonella cholerae-suis was first isolated and carefully studied by Salmon and Smith (21) in 1885. They spoke of it as the bacillus of hog cholera, but hog cholera is now recognized as a virus disease. Other synonyms are *B. cholerae-suis*, Smith, 1893, 1894; *B. choleraesuum*, Migula, 1895 (Engler and Prantl, 1895); *B. suipestifer*, Kruse, 1896 (Flugge, 1896); *B. salmoni*, Chester, 1901. The antigenic structure (5) is VI, VII:c:1, 5.

Salmonella cholerae-suis has been found on rare occasions to cause serious human infections (20). The natural and only host appears to be the pig.

Salmonella meleagridis was first described by Bruner and Edwards (106) after isolation from turkey poults in Minnesota. They (42) reported it in fowl, swine, and man. It has a wide geographic distribution. The antigenic formula is III, X, XXVI:e, h:l, w.

Salmonella anatum was first isolated from ducklings in a case of mixed infection with *S. typhimurium* and *S. newington*. It has been found in many parts of the world. It has the following antigenic formula: III, X, XXVI:e, h:l, 6. . . .

Salmonella panama was isolated by Jordan (107) from an outbreak characterized by symptoms of dizziness, headache, and nausea (rarely vomiting), followed later by diarrhea and fever in about 40 men belonging to two batteries of American soldiers in the Panama Canal Zone. The food suspected was meat hash that had been served in the morning. Illness began to develop in the evening, although 2 of the men did not feel ill until the following morning. The natural habitat of *S. panama* is unknown. Since Jordan's report, 4 cases (108) in infants have been described, 2 of which were fatal. The antigenic structure (5) of *S. panama* is I, IX, XII:l, v:1, 5. . . .

Many more species or types of *Salmonella* than the few listed have been implicated in gastrointestinal disturbances in man. As pointed out in the first part of the chapter, the pathogenicity for different individuals varies widely, even with well-recognized types. There appears to be similar variability in pathogenicity for animals. For example, *S. aberdeen, S. give, S. california, S. worthington, S. orani-*

enburg, S. paratyphi B, *S. new brunswick, S. urbana, S. hvittingfoss, S. muenchen,* and *S. pullorum* (109) were isolated from the intestinal contents or feces of chickens, and subcultures in veal-infusion broth containing 1 per cent starch were fed in 50-ml. quantities to *Macaca mulatta.* None of the animals developed any symptoms or signs of illness. Furthermore, viscera of swine (110), mainly cecum and colon from 16 different field cases of nondysentery enteritis, were fed to 27 cholera-vaccinated shotes without causing any significant effect. Living *S. cholerae-suis* was present in at least 8 of the viscera which were fed to cholera-vaccinated pigs with negative results.

Hormaeche, Peluffo, and Aleppo (111) called attention to the greater susceptibility of young children to *Salmonella* infections. Five human volunteers (112) were fed from 2,000,000,000 to 4,-000,000,000 organisms of a strain of *S. typhimurium* isolated from a fatal case of a 6-month-old child and developed mild to fairly severe reactions of not more than 3 days' duration.

Obviously, many of the well-recognized species or types of *Salmonella* may cause gastrointestinal disturbances, and more critical study is needed before the pathogenicity for man of some of the less common may be properly evaluated. *Salmonella* are inhabitants of the intestinal tract of man and animals, and several species have been isolated from the stools of healthy men and animals. It is important that other causative agents be excluded in cases of gastrointestinal disturbances when evaluating the significance of a *Salmonella* type found in the stools. Recently, *S. pullorum* (65) was implicated in an outbreak of gastroenteritis involving a known total of 423 persons, of whom 172 were hospitalized. *Salmonella pullorum,* isolated from the stools of 11.7 per cent of the hospitalized patients, was believed to have been the probable cause of the infection. As pointed out elsewhere (113), no food items were available for bacteriological examination. Furthermore, the investigation was made after the peak of the epidemic and during the convalescence of the patients. No report was made of a search for other agents. Another work (114) appeared in which *S. pullorum* was isolated from the stools of a patient at the onset of diarrhea. Since man has been eating raw or incompletely cooked eggs for centuries, it appears unusual that infections with *S. pullorum* should not have been discovered before the present reports.

As study of the pathogenicity of the enteric group of bacilli progresses, it is obvious that it forms a gradient series of microörganisms with the more highly pathogenic typhoid and dysentery group at one extreme, grading down through the *Salmonella* and paracolon groups to the less pathogenic colon aerogenes group at the other extreme.

The detailed serological procedure for the identification of species is apt to lead to confusion unless it is carefully supervised. Simplified routine typing methods have been developed for use in diagnostic laboratories (45).

REFERENCES

1. SALMON, DANIEL E., and SMITH, THEOBALD. Rep. Com. Agr., Washington, D.C., 1885, 1886.
2. KAUFFMANN, F. Enterobacteriaceae. Kopenhagen: Einar Munksgaard, 1951.
3. VOLLUM, R. L., and TAYLOR, JOAN. Medical Research Council, Spec. Rep. Ser., No. 260, pp. 29–31. London: H.M. Stationery Office, 1947.
4. JORDAN, E. O., and HARMON, P. H. J. Infect. Dis., 42:238, 1928.
5. KAUFFMANN, F. Die Bakteriologie der Salmonella-Gruppe. Kopenhagen: Einar Munksgaard, 1941.
6. Medical Research Council, Spec. Rep. Ser., No. 103, 1926.
7. Rep. Proc., 3d Internat. Cong. Microbiol., September 2–9, 1939, pp. 833–40. New York, 1940.
8. EDWARDS, P. R., and BRUNER, D. W. Kentucky Agr. Exper. Stat. Circ., 54, 1, 1942.
9. EDWARDS, P. R., and MORAN, ALICE B. Proc. Soc. Exper. Biol. & Med., 61:242–43, 1946.
10. BRUNER, D. W., and EDWARDS, P. R. J. Bact., 55:449, 1948.
11. GÄRTNER, A. Korresp. d. allg. ärztl. Ver. Thüringen, 17:233, 1888.
12. ERMENGEM, E. VAN. Rev. d'hyg., 18:761–819, 1896.
13. DAUER, C. C. Pub. Health Rep., 67:1093–94, 1952.
14. ————. *Ibid.*, 68:700–701, 1953.
15. DAUER, C. C., and SYLVESTER, G. Pub. Health Rep., 69:541, 1954.
16. FELSENFELD, OSCAR, YOUNG, VIOLA MAE, and YOSHIMURA, TAMA. Am. J. Digest. Dis., 18:209–13, 1951.
17. Month. Bull. Min. Health, 9:254, 1950.
    Ibid., 10:228–39, 1951.
    COCKBURN, W. C. Personal communication.
18. ROSENAU, M. J., and WEISS, H. J.A.M.A., 77:1948–50, 1921.
19. SPRAY, R. S. J.A.M.A., 86:109–11, 1926.
20. STEWART, H. C., and LITTERER, WILLIAM. J.A.M.A., 89:1584–87, 1927.

21. SCHYTTE, BLIX A., and TESDAL, MARTIN. Norsk mag. lægevidensk., **89:** 689–709, 1928.
22. CULLEY, A. R. Brit. M. J., **1:**325, 1937.
23. BROWN, EARLE G., COMBS, G. R., and WRIGHT, EVAN. J.A.M.A., **114:** 642–44, 1940.
24. HAUSER, GEORGE H., TREUTING, W. L., and BREIFFELH, L. A. Pub. Health Rep., **60:**1138–42, 1945.
25. PERCH, BEATE. Acta pathol. et microbiol. scandinav., **24:**399–400, 1947.
26. EDWARDS, P. R. Personal communication.
27. DACK, G. M., and DAVISON, ELLEN. Food Res., **3:**347–49, 1938.
28. DACK, G. M. J. Am. Vet. M. A., **97:**123–24, 1940.
29. SAVAGE, WILLIAM G., and WHITE, P. BRUCE. Medical Research Council, Rep. No. 92. London: H.M. Stationery Office, 1925.
30. ———. Medical Research Council, Rep. No. 91. London, 1925.
31. BRANHAM, SARA ELIZABETH. J. Infect. Dis., **37:**291–308, 1925.
32. BAHR, L., and DYSSEGAARD, A. Centralbl. f. Bakt., **102:**268, 1927.
33. DACK, GAIL M., CARY, WILLIAM E., and HARMON, PAUL H. J. Prevent. Med., **2:**479–83, 1928.
34. GEIGER, J. C., and MEYER, K. F. Proc. Soc. Exper. Biol. & Med., **26:** 91, 1928.
35. BRANHAM, SARA E., ROBEY, LUCILE, and DAY, LOIS A. J. Infect. Dis., **43:**507–15, 1928.
36. SAVAGE, WILLIAM G. J. Hyg., **33:**233–44, 1933.
37. DACK, GAIL M., HARMON, PAUL H., and JARRA, IRENE E. J. Prevent. Med., **2:**461–78, 1928.
38. ELKELES, G. Ergebn. Hyg., Bakt., **11:**68, 1930.
39. DACK, G. M., JORDAN, E. O., and WOOD, W. L. J. Prevent. Med., **3:** 153–58, 1929.
40. VERDER, ELIZABETH, and SUTTON, CHARLES. J. Infect. Dis., **53:**262–71, 1933.
41. HAMMERSCHMIDT, J. Wein. klin. Wchnschr., **48:**325–30, 1935.
42. EDWARDS, P. R., and BRUNER, D. W. J. Infect. Dis., **72:**58–67, 1943.
43. BORNSTEIN, S., SAPHRA, I., and STRAUSS, L. J. Infect. Dis., **69:**59–64, 1941.
44. BORMAN, EARLE K., WHEELER, KENNETH M., WEST, D. EVELYN, and MICKLE, FRIEND LEE. Am. J. Pub. Health, **33:**127–34, 1943.
45. LINDBERG, ROBERT B., and BAYLISS, MILWARD. J. Infect. Dis., **79:**91–95, 1946.
46. HENDERSON, LOWELL L. Am. J. Trop. Med., **27:**643–55, 1947.
47. BOYER, J., and TISSIER, MLLE. Presse méd., **57:**1028–30, 1949.
48. BRUNER, D. W., and MORAN, ALICE B. Cornell Vet., **39:**53–63, 1949.
49. MACKEL, DON C., GALTON, MILDRED M., GRAY, HERMAN, and HARDY, ALBERT V. J. Infect. Dis., **91:**15–18, 1952.
50. WOLFF, ARTHUR H., HENDERSON, NORMAN D., and McCALLUM, GRACE L. Am. J. Pub. Health, **38:**403–8, 1948.
51. STUCKER, CALVIN L., GALTON, MILDRED M., COWDERY, JOHN, and HARDY, ALBERT V. J. Infect. Dis., **91:**6–11, 1952.
52. HINSHAW, W. R., McNEIL, E., and TAYLOR, T. J. Am. J. Hyg., **40:** 264–78, 1944.

53. EDWARDS, P. R., BRUNER, D. W., and MORAN, ALICE B. Cornell Vet., **38**:247–56, 1948.
54. CORPRON, RUTH, BIVINS, J. A., and STAFSETH, H. J. Poultry Sc., **26**: 340–51, 1947.
55. GAUMONT, R. Ann. Inst. Pasteur, **3**:140, 1950.
56. SMITH, H. WILLIAMS, and BUXTON, A. Brit. M. J., **1**:1478, 1951.
57. HEMMES, G. D. Overdruk Uit "Geneeskundige Gids," March 6, 1952.
58. MILNER, KELSEY C., and SHAFFER, MORRIS F. J. Infect. Dis., **90**:81–96, 1952.
59. HUSSEMAN, DOROTHY L., and WALLACE, MARGARET A. Food Res., **16**: 89–96, 1951.
60. WATT, JAMES. Pub. Health Rep., **60**:835–39, 1945.
61. SCOTT, W. M. Bull. Office internat. d'hyg. pub., **25**:828–33, 1933.
62. GERNEZ-RIEUX, C., BUTTIAUX, R., KESTELOOT, A., and SUFFRAN, R. Presse méd., **35**:479, 1949.
63. McCULLOUGH, NORMAN B., and EISELE, C. WESLEY. J. Infect. Dis., **89**:209–13, 1951.
64. Quoted from EDWARDS, P. R. Proc. 7th World Poultry Cong., p. 271, 1939.
65. MITCHELL, ROLAND B., GARLOCK, FRED C., and BROH-KAHN, R. H. J. Infect. Dis., **79**:57–62, 1946.
66. CARTER, MARY JUNE, POWELL, MARCUS P., and BORTS, IRVING H. Pub. Health Rep., **65**:778–81, 1950.
67. BERNSTEIN, A. Month. Bull. Min. Health, **11**:64–67, 1952.
68. GIBBONS, N. E., and MOORE, R. L. Canad. J. Res. (F), **22**:48–57, 1944.
69. SOLOWEY, MATHILDE, McFARLANE, VERNON H., SPAULDING, E. H., and CHEMERDA, CECILIA. Am. J. Pub. Health, **37**:971–82, 1947.
70. OLIN, GUNNAR. Personal communication, letter dated 4/23/54.
71. SOLOWEY, MATHILDE, and CALESNICK, ELEANOR J. Food Res., **13**:216–26, 1948.
72. GORESLINE, HARRY E., HAYES, KIRBY M., MOSER, ROY E., HOWE, MILTON A., JR., and DREWNIAK, EDWIN E. U.S. Dept. Agr., Circ. No. 897, October, 1951.
73. WINTER, A. R. Food Technol., **6**:414–15, 1952.
74. ANELLIS, A., LUBAS, J., and RAYMAN, MORTON M. Food Technol., Vol. **6**, No. 5, abstr. from 12th annual meeting, 1952.
75. OSBORNE, W. W., STRAKA, R. P., and LINEWEAVER, HANS. Food Technol., Vol. **6**, No. 5, abstr. from 12th annual meeting, 1952.
76. AYRES, JOHN C. Food Technol., **3**:172–76, 1949.
77. CLINGER, CAROLINE, YOUNG, ARLENE, PRUDENT, INEZ, and WINTER, A. R. Food Technol., **5**:166–70, 1951.
78. AYRES, JOHN C., and SLOSBERG, H. M. Food Technol., **3**:180–83, 1949.
79. HORMAECHE, E., and SALSAMENDI, R. Arch. urug. med., **9**:665–72, 1936.
80. RUBIN, H. L., SCHERAGO, M., and WEAVER, R. H. Am. J. Hyg., **36**: 43–47, 1942.
81. KRANEVELD, F. C., ERBER, M., and MANSJOER, M. Hemera zoa, **58**: 48–73, 1951.

82. CLARENBURG, A., VINK, H. H., and HUISMAN, W. Antonie van Leeuwenhoek, **15**:14–16, 1949.
83. GAUMONT, R. Ann. Inst. Pasteur, **5**:177–90, 1952–53.
84. KÄMPE, A., LILLEENGEN, K., and ÖSTERLING, S. Nord. vet., **6**:190–95, 1951.
85. GALTON, MILDRED M., SMITH W. V., McELRATH, HUNTER B., and HARDY, A. V. J. Infect. Dis., **95**:236–45, 1954.
86. GALTON, MILDRED M., LOWERY, WILLA DEAN, and HARDY, ALBERT V. J. Infect. Dis., **95**:232–35, 1954.
87. LILLEENGEN, K., and MICKOW, R. Nord. vet. med., **4**:127–32, 1952.
88. CHERRY, W. B., SCHERAGO, M., and WEAVER, R. H. Am. J. Hyg., **37**: 211–15, 1943.
89. BARTRAM, M. T., WELCH, H., and OSTROLENK, M. J. Infect. Dis., **67**: 222–26, 1940.
90. WELCH, HENRY, OSTROLENK, M., and BARTRAM, M. T. Am. J. Pub. Health, **31**:332–40, 1941.
91. AUSTEN, F. E. J. Roy. Army M. Corps, **2**:651, 1904.
92. NORTH CAROLINA BOARD OF HEALTH. Spec. Bull. 8, June, 1912.
93. OSTROLENK, M., and WELCH, H. Am. J. Pub. Health, **32**:487–94, 1942.
94. ESKEY, C. R., PRINCE, FRANK M., and FULLER, FRANK B. Pub. Health Rep., **64**:933–41, 1949.
95. OLSON, THEODORE A., and RUEGER, MYRTLE E. Pub. Health Rep., **65**: 531–40, 1950.
96. SEGALOVE, MILTON, and DACK, G. M. Food Res., **9**:1–5, 1944.
97. McCULLOUGH, NORMAN B., and EISELE, C. WESLEY. J. Infect. Dis., **88**:278–89, 1951.
98. ———. *Ibid.*, **89**:259–65, 1951.
99. ———. J. Immunol., **66**:595–608, 1951.
100. McCULLOUGH, NORMAN B. Pub. Health Rep., **66**:1538–40, 1951.
101. Diagnostic procedures and reagents. 3d ed. New York: American Public Health Association, 1950.
102. U.S. Public Health Service, National Office of Vital Statistics, communicable disease summary for week ended January 3, 1953.
103. SCHÜTZE, H. Lancet, **1**:93, 1920.
104. KAUFFMANN, F. Ztschr. Hyg., **111**:221–32, 1930.
105. HORMAECHE, E., and PELUFFO, C. A. Arch. urug. med., **9**:673–76, 1936.
106. BRUNER, D. W., and EDWARDS, P. R. Am. J. Hyg., B, **34**:82–86, 1941.
107. JORDAN, EDWIN O. J. Infect. Dis., **55**:224–27, 1934.
108. SCHIFF, FRITZ. J.A.M.A., **111**:2458–60, 1938.
109. MALLMANN, W. L., RYFF, J. F., and MATTHEWS, EVELYN. J. Infect. Dis., **70**:253–62, 1942.
110. DOYLE, L. P., and WALKEY, F. L. J. Am. Vet. M. A., **109**:280–82, 1946.
111. HORMAECHE, E., PELUFFO, C. A., and ALEPPO, P. L. Arch. pediat., Uruguay, **11**:8–28, 1940.
112. ———. Arch. urug. med., **9**:113–62, 1936.
113. DACK, G. M. Am. J. Pub. Health, **37**:360–64, 1947.
114. JUDEFIND, T. F. J. Bact., **54**:667, 1947.

VII Streptococcus faecalis in Relation to Food Poisoning

Alpha-type streptococci grew readily on the surface of blood agar plates. Around the minute pinpoint colonies a greenish zone develops, owing to the chemical change in the hemoglobin, and this is the basis for the classification "alpha type" (1). Many workers (2, 3, 4) have considered α-type streptococci responsible for food-poisoning outbreaks when they were predominant in suspected foods, even where no illness was caused when they were fed to animals. Linden, Turner, and Thom (5), however, actually observed symptoms of food poisoning in cats that were fed living cultures of streptococci isolated during an outbreak. Unfortunately, the reactions of experimental animals may not be the same as man's. The α-type streptococcus strain was studied a number of years later by Sherman, Smiley, and Niven (6) and was found to be *Streptococcus faecalis*, belonging to the Lancefield serological group D.

In our laboratory, 4 outbreaks in which α-type streptococci predominated in the incriminated food were studied bacteriologically. In 2 of these outbreaks, involving canned Vienna sausage (7) and beef croquettes (8), cultures of the organisms and filtrates were studied in human volunteers. The other 2 incidents implicated coconut cream pie and turkey dressing (not previously reported). In the first outbreak, 75 out of 182 boys had eaten a Sunday evening meal at which Vienna sausages were served. Other foods and water were ruled out on epidemiological grounds. The sausages were taken from 6 large (No. 10) cans and were served without heating. They had no abnormal appearance, odor, or taste. Since less than half the boys became ill, and only 1 of 4 unopened cans contained the organisms, it is probable that only 1 or 2 cans were contaminated. The symptoms included nausea, vomiting, colic-like pains, and diarrhea. Most of the boys became ill within 4–5 hours, although a few did not begin to exhibit symptoms until 12 hours after supper. All recovered within 24 hours after the onset of symptoms.

Three sausages left from the supper were examined bacteriologically and found to contain large numbers of slowly growing, pleomorphic, α-type streptococci. These organisms in veal-infusion broth cultures were readily killed when heated to 60° C. for 1 hour or 85° C. for 15 minutes. No *Salmonella* were found. Four unopened cans of sausage, with the same code markings, were later examined. One can contained viable organisms essentially identical with those isolated from the sausages remaining from supper. The unopened can in which the contaminated sausages were found showed defective seams, through which the streptococci may have entered. When cultures from this can had been incubated for 4 days, before growth was evident, a young adult laboratory worker ate half a sausage from each of the 4 cans. Five hours later she developed nausea, which increased for 24 hours, with two periods of vomiting accompanied by epigastric pain and exhaustion. A second volunteer drank 40 ml. of a 5-day beef heart culture and became ill 5 hours later. Belching was followed in 24 hours by unsuccessful attempts at vomiting, intermittent epigastric pain, tenesmus, cold perspiration, temperature of 99°2 F., and marked exhaustion. A third volunteer drank 50 ml. of a bacteria-free filtrate prepared from a similar culture and suffered no ill effects. Mice, guinea pigs, rabbits, and monkeys (*Macaca mulatta*) were fed cultures of these streptococci but showed no symptoms. Three young cats which were fed 48-hour milk cultures had soft stools the following day but otherwise appeared to be unaffected.

The outbreak involving croquettes (fried minced-meat balls with rice and egg) occurred in a group of 250 men between seventeen and twenty-five years of age. The noon meal was found on epidemiological evidence to have been responsible. Samples of all remaining foods were sent to the laboratory 2 days later. Both epidemiological and laboratory evidence showed that the beef croquettes, which were prepared from beef stew, round of beef, and Swedish meat balls remaining from the meal of the preceding evening, were implicated. These were put into a large container and were left covered at room temperature until the following morning, when they were placed in the refrigerator until time for preparation. They were chopped together mechanically and mixed with bread crumbs and gravy made 2 days previously. Then they were fried in deep fat at about 110°

C. for 10 minutes while the meal was being served and apparently tasted satisfactory, since several second helpings were eaten. Conditions in the kitchen were sanitary, and no rat or vermin poisons were recently used. The kitchen employees were given routine health examinations. However, the cook had a head cold on the day that the croquettes were served.

By the questionnaire method, information was obtained from 208 of the men, 117 of whom were made ill. Sixty-three of the 91 who were not ill ate croquettes. This fact may have been due to their high resistance or to a variation in the time of frying the croquettes. Among the 117 who were ill, 98 reported that they had eaten the croquettes. Since the questionnaire was circulated nearly a week after the outbreak, some discrepancies in reporting were to be expected. Diarrhea—the outstanding symptom—was reported in 110 cases, 3 reported vomiting, 15 nausea, and 55 abdominal cramps. The incubation period was from 6 to 18 hours in 104 individuals and was generally about 12 hours. In 3, it was 3 hours or less. The symptoms subsided in from 6 to 24 hours in all cases except 4, where they persisted for over 3 days. It is obvious that this outbreak was unusually mild and consisted essentially in the development of diarrhea after an incubation period of several hours.

No *Salmonella* were found in specimens of the food, but numerous α-type streptococci were present on the blood agar plates. Five days after the outbreak, a weighed sample of the refrigerated croquettes was ground with sterile sand, taken up in saline, and plated in decimal dilutions in blood agar. After the culture had grown for 24 hours, a plate count of 280,000,000 green-producing streptococci was found per gram. This was not an accurate count, because the streptococci were clumped, and the laboratory test was not made immediately after the outbreak. Seven volunteers between the ages of twenty-two and thirty years, who were not subject to spontaneous gastrointestinal disturbances, drank milk to which had been added varying amounts up to 20 ml. of the filtrate of the culture grown in veal-infusion broth. None was made ill. Five volunteers felt abdominal distress after taking broth cultures containing living streptococci one or more times.

From these outbreaks it can be seen that, although α-type streptococci may give rise to symptoms of food poisoning in man, culture filtrates of these organisms will not do so.

The outbreak caused by turkey dressing occurred at a banquet at which three-quarters of 393 people who were served were made ill. Fifteen or sixteen fresh turkeys were stuffed in one evening, placed in the refrigerator overnight, roasted from 8:00 A.M. to 1:30 or 2:00 P.M. on the following day, left in open pans to cool, carved at 4:30 P.M., and placed atop the range in open pans until they were served. The meal was eaten between 8:30 and 9:00 P.M. in the evening (5–6 hours later), and illness began to occur at approximately 4:00 A.M. the next morning and continued until noon. The incubation period was from 7 to 15 hours. The symptoms consisted generally of abdominal cramping and diarrhea, with some nausea, vomiting, and prostration. Blood agar plates streaked with a suspension of either the turkey or the turkey dressing and incubated for 24 hours at 37° C. contained numerous colonies of α-type streptococci in almost pure culture. A study of this strain by Buchbinder *et al.* (9) showed it to be *S. faecalis.* No *Salmonella* were found on plates of eosin–methylene blue agar streaked with the specimen.

Streptococcus faecalis was found in samples of dried eggs which are known to be toxic to man when eaten (10), as well as in many samples of dried egg not known to be toxic. A 10 per cent suspension of dried egg in quarter-strength Ringer's solution was heated in a 70° C. water bath for 1 hour for three periods, each followed by a 3–6-hour interval of incubation at 37° C. After the last heating period, 50-ml. quantities were inoculated with 1/50–1/25 ml. of a $1\frac{1}{2}$–$2\frac{1}{2}$-hour actively growing culture of *S. faecalis.* The egg cultures were incubated for 24–48 hours, with final colony counts of 100,000,-000–750,000,000 organisms per milliliter. Ten-milliliter portions heated in a 70° C. water bath for 45 minutes were fed to 5 human volunteers without producing ill effects.

Buchbinder and his co-workers (9) reported bacteriological studies and other pertinent data in 4 outbreaks of food poisoning, in which enterococci were the predominant organisms isolated from the suspected foods (canned evaporated milk, charlotte russe, roast beef, and ham bologna).

In the outbreak involving evaporated milk, the cans were from a lot canned 2 years previously and stored or handled under conditions causing spoilage; many cans were rusty, leakers, springers, or swells. There were 74 out of 161 children ill within 2–7 hours after a meal. Symptoms were characterized by abdominal cramps, nausea, and vomiting. Diarrhea was reported in only 2 cases. All the children were symptom-free within 6 hours after the onset of illness. Mashed potatoes and pasteurized milk were the only foods common to those who became ill. Unfortunately, since none of the implicated foods was examined, the evidence was circumstantial. Heat-stable staphylococcus enterotoxin in the absence of viable staphylococci was not excluded as a cause of this outbreak, which took place in a children's institution.

The outbreak involving charlotte russe concerned 3 members of a family who became ill within $5\frac{1}{2}$–12 hours after eating the cake. Symptoms consisted of abdominal cramps, vomiting, and diarrhea. The charlotte russe was the only food eaten in common. Specimens of the ingredients used were obtained from the bakery and consisted of sponge cake, gelatin, skimmed condensed milk, and whipped cream. The sponge cake contained only about 800 bacteria per gram, which were almost entirely coliform organisms. The gelatin contained 3×10^5 organisms per gram, although prior to its use in the pastry it had been heated in a double boiler for 15–18 hours. A bacterial count of 54,000 organisms per milliliter was present in the skimmed condensed milk, mostly enterococci. The whipped cream yielded a total of 1×10^7 organisms per gram, which were largely *S. faecalis*.

The outbreak implicating barbecued beef involved a group of people who had attended a wedding anniversary dinner. The incubation period was generally 10–12 hours, the extremes being 3 and 15 hours. Symptoms were mild, a few individuals were nauseated and vomited, whereas the majority experienced only abdominal cramping and diarrhea. Seventy-four out of 87 persons interviewed had become ill. The meat had been roasted over hickory logs on the evening before it was consumed and had been left unrefrigerated in the roasting room of the delicatessen from 10:30 P.M. until 11:00 A.M. the following morning. About 50 pounds were then sliced and taken to a synagogue, where they remained unrefrigerated until 3:00 P.M. At that time the meat was placed in pans and heated in a slow oven for 1 hour and was eaten at 4:00–5:00 P.M. Samples of the meat and of the gravy, made from turkey and chicken drippings, served with the meat were taken from refrigerators, where the left-over food had been placed following the dinner. A count of 4.5 × 10^6 organisms per gram, with enterococci predominating, was found for the meat and 1×10^5 to 2.4×10^5 per milliliter for the gravy.

The ham bologna involved in the fourth outbreak was part of one shipment distributed by a large chain retail grocery company to a number of its stores in the New York City metropolitan area. The company had been notified of additional outbreaks outside the city and had recalled the meat. Nine persons from 3 families ate the ham. Symptoms began in 3–6 hours and lasted from 3 to 48 hours. These consisted of vomiting, abdominal cramps, and diarrhea. A count of 3.5×10^6 organisms per gram, mainly *S. faecalis,* was found.

Experimental studies have been carried out in which the α-type streptococcus (*S. faecalis* from the outbreak implicating the turkey dressing discussed) was inoculated into various types of canned goods (11). The organism was demonstrated for at least 30 days at 37° C. in canned foods of low-acid content (corn, peas), semiacid content (asparagus, spinach, string beans), a highly acid product (tomato juice), and sea food (shrimp and salmon). Organisms were demonstrable in all cases for 60 days at 22° and at 37° C. in most instances. Growth did not occur in sugar-preserved canned peaches (a highly acid product); and viable organisms were not cultured after 2 days. Although α-type streptococci are killed by the time and temperature used in processing canned foods, the ability of these organisms to grow and survive in these products is of practical importance to the problem of food poisoning. Contamination of the contents of a can with these organisms may occur after the can is opened, after which storage at temperatures supporting growth might lead to the development of large numbers of organisms capable of giving rise to gastrointestinal symptoms on ingestion. The physiological characteristics (12) of *S. faecalis* are such that it may well find conditions in the opened can of food suitable for multiplication. For example, *S. faecalis* is characterized by its ability to grow fairly rapidly over a wide temperature range (10°–45° C.) or to grow in salt concentrations of 6.5 per cent and higher and, finally, by its heat resistance, to survive the time and temperature of pasteurization.

Moore (13) described an outbreak in five different schools, involving children who had only one meal in common. Chocolate pudding was found to be responsible for the outbreak. It had been stored under time and temperature conditions which permitted bacterial multiplication. Alpha-hemolytic streptococci were isolated in large numbers from the pudding and were the only bacteria found. Living cultures and culture filtrates of this streptococcus produced food-poisoning symptoms in a human volunteer similar to those reported in the outbreak and occurred after a similar incubation period. The incubation periods in a group of 41 children in one school are given in the accompanying table. The species identifica-

Incubation Period (Hours)	No. of Children	Incubation Period (Hours)	No. of Children
3	1	14–16	8
5–7	6	17–19	3
8–10	7	20–22	1
11–13	15		

tion of the streptococcus studied by Moore was not definitely established. He suggests that Cary *et al.* (7, 8) might have found filtrates toxic if they had used a medium other than veal-infusion broth.

Dack, Niven, Kirsner, and Marshall (14) fed human volunteers a specific strain of *S. faecalis* which was used as a starter culture for cheese. Since *S. faecalis* decarboxylates tyrosine to produce tyramine, the effect of feeding tyramine to human volunteers was also tested. Cheese made with the starter strain of *S. faecalis*, which contained large numbers of viable organisms as well as appreciable quantities of tyramine, was without effect when fed to human volunteers. Tyramine monohydrochloride, in 0.3- or 1-gm. amounts, when fed to human volunteers in 1 pint of milk, caused no rise in blood pressure or other ill effects. In 2 and possibly 3 volunteers, illness occurred after the feeding of a milk culture of a strain of *S. liquefaciens* recently isolated from an outbreak of food poisoning. The illness consisted of nausea and diarrheal stools of short duration, beginning 32–36 hours after the test feeding. Two strains of *S. faecalis* isolated from other outbreaks were without effect when similarly fed to human volunteers. These experiments involved 52 feeding tests on 37 volunteers. The reason for the negative tests with strains of *S. faecalis* is not apparent. Factors to be considered may be that the strains underwent change upon laboratory cultivation, or perhaps positive results might have been obtained if the strains had been grown in sterilized foods other than milk as culture media. Cheddar cheese under the conditions of the reported experiments was not a medium suitable for causing food-poisoning illnesses with the strain of *S. faecalis* tested.

TABLE 13

CHARACTERISTICS OF FOOD POISONING CAUSED
BY BACTERIA OR THEIR PRODUCTS

Disease	Specific Agent	Intoxication	Infection	Symptoms	Onset of Symptoms after Eating
Botulism	*Clostridium botulinum,* which produces toxin	+	−	Difficulty in swallowing, double vision (diplopia), difficulty in speech (aphonia), difficulty in respiration, followed by death from paralysis of muscles of respiration	2 hours–8 days; average 1–2 days
Staphylococcus food poisoning	Staphylococci which produce enterotoxin	+	−	Nausea, vomiting, diarrhea, and acute prostration; abdominal cramps	1–6 hours; average 2½–3 hours
Salmonella infection	*S. typhimurium; S. enteritidis; S. cholerae-suis*	−	+	Abdominal pain, diarrhea, chills, fever, frequent vomiting, prostration	7–72 hours
Streptococcus food poisoning	α-type (*S. faecalis*)	−	+	Nausea, sometimes vomiting, colicky pains, and diarrhea	2–18 hours
Bacillus cereus food poisoning	*Bacillus cereus*	−	+		
Clostridium perfringens food poisoning	*Clostridium perfringens*	−	+		

More study of *S. faecalis* is needed to explain many of the puzzling problems in which this organism is implicated in gastrointestinal illness. Every year additional outbreaks are reported, although their number is small when compared to staphylococcus food poisoning. Laboratory experiments in feeding cultures to human volunteers have not led to clear-cut results, such as characterize outbreaks in which the majority of a group of people is ill after the consumption of a food containing large numbers of *S. faecalis,* which is a natural inhabitant of the bowel. However, unusually large numbers in some foods may cause illness. Where human volunteers are fed cultures to be tested for pathogenicity, better results may be obtained if, instead of feeding broth cultures, the organisms were grown in foods identical to those involved in an outbreak.

The incubation period from the time of eating food contaminated with α-type streptococci to the onset of illness, which is longer than that of staphylococcus food-poisoning outbreaks, varies from 2 to 18 hours. In children the incubation period may be shorter than in adults. Symptoms of this type of food poisoning are usually milder than in staphylococcus food poisoning, and the beginning of illness is spread out over a length of time. This longer period appears to occur when living agents are involved, as in *S. faecalis* and *Salmonella* infections of the food-poisoning type, whereas a shorter one occurs if enterotoxin is responsible (cf. Table 13). As stated previously, the longer incubation period may represent the time required for multiplication of the organisms in the intestinal tract before the infection manifests itself.

Sherman and his co-workers (15) should be credited with recognizing that the streptococci implicated in food poisoning fall into one species. They found that a total of six strains of nonhemolytic streptococci isolated by others from an equal number of outbreaks were *S. faecalis.* Perhaps only a small quantity of *S. faecalis* strains causes gastrointestinal symptoms. Future work is needed to settle this problem. Certainly, the species is a natural inhabitant of the intestinal tract of man and animals and, as a consequence, is in man's food and drink. In all outbreaks of streptococcus food poisoning large numbers of the organisms are ingested in the implicated foods, and dosage undoubtedly plays a role in the initiation of illness.

REFERENCES

1. BROWN, J. H. Monogr. Rockefeller Inst. M. Res., No. 9, 1919.
2. New York State Health News, 1:51, 1924; 5:206, 1928.
3. AOKI, K., and SAKAI, K. Centralbl. f. Bakt., Abt. 1, 98:145, 1926.
4. NELSON, N. A. New England J. Med., 199:1145–48, 1928.
5. LINDEN, B. A., TURNER, W. R., and THOM, CHARLES. Pub. Health Rep., 41:1647–52, 1926.

6. SHERMAN, J. M., SMILEY, KARL L., and NIVEN, CHARLES F., JR., J. Dairy Sc., **26**:321–23, 1943.
7. CARY, W. E., DACK, G. M., and MYERS, ELIZABETH. Proc. Soc. Exper. Biol. & Med., **29**:214–15, 1931.
8. CARY, WILLIAM E., DACK, G. M., and DAVISON, ELLEN. J. Infect. Dis., **62**:88–91, 1938.
9. BUCHBINDER, L., OSLER, A. G., and STEFFEN, G. I. Pub. Health Rep., **63**:109–18, 1948.
10. TOPLEY, ELIZABETH. Medical Research Council, Spec. Rep. Ser., No. 260, pp. 53–57. London: H. M. Stationery Office, 1947.
11. SURGALLA, MICHAEL, SEGALOVE, MILTON, and DACK, G. M. Food Res., **9**:112–14, 1944.
12. SHERMAN, JAMES M. Bact. Rev., **1**:1–97, 1937.
13. MOORE, B. Month. Bull. Min. Health, pp. 136–44, June, 1948.
14. DACK, G. M., NIVEN, C. F., JR., KIRSNER, J. B., and MARSHALL, HOMER. J. Infect. Dis., **85**:131–38, 1949.
15. SHERMAN, J. M., GUNSALUS, I. C., and BELLAMY, W. D. 57th ann. rep., New York State Coll. Agr., Cornell Univ. Agr. Exper. Stat., p. 116, 1944.

VIII Significance of Other Bacteria in Food Poisoning

Microörganisms other than those previously referred to have been implicated in outbreaks of food poisoning, but the evidence incriminating them is not conclusive. An interesting example can be cited from studies of water-borne outbreaks of typhoid fever. When water is contaminated suddenly with sewage, cases showing symptoms of diarrhea, abdominal cramping, and nausea frequently occur within 12–48 hours. This relationship, shown by Jordan and Irons (1) in an outbreak in Rockford, Illinois, in 1912 is well summarized in a report on a subsequent outbreak occurring in another city. The authors make the following statement:

> Thus in the Rockford epidemic, due to a sudden and temporary pollution of the water supply by sewage, the probable number of cases of initial enteritis was over 10,000 in a population of 50,000 but careful search for cases of typhoid revealed only about 200 cases. Out of the total of 46 persons residing in one block, 44 drank sufficient water to produce gastro-intestinal disturbance, in some instances, mild with little or no diarrhea, in others, very severe with nausea, vomiting, purging and marked prostration, and yet only one person of the 44 suffered from typhoid fever later [2].

A similar example came to the author's attention in 1934, when there was a large fire in the Chicago Stock Yards. Much water was pumped from the mains, and sewage gained entrance to the water of the district from a drainage ditch. After 8 hours or more, a number of individuals who drank from the hydrants in the area suffered acute gastrointestinal upsets. Symptoms were mild and disappeared in a few days. Nevertheless, in due course of time, several cases of typhoid fever and amebic dysentery occurred among the populace drinking the contaminated water. The cause of acute gastrointestinal disturbances which follow drinking sewage-polluted water after a few hours has not been established but may be a specific pathogenic microörganism.

Escherichia coli

A specific strain of *Escherichia coli* was isolated by Bray (3) from infant diarrhea and named *Bacterium coli* var. *neapolitanum*. The same type was isolated from infant diarrhea in Scotland by Giles and Sangster (4). Giles, Sangster, and Smith (5) called their strain *B. coli alpha*. One isolated from infant diarrhea in England by Taylor, Powell, and Wright (6) was called *B. coli* D433. These strains described under various names were found to be identical. With Kauffmann's classification (7), all the types fall into one of two groups, either 0111B$_4$ or 055B$_5$. Smith, Galloway, and Speirs (8) have tabulated the strains according to authors and designations given.

Neter and co-workers (9) fed a strain of *E. coli* serotype 0111 (D433) to a two-month-old infant who had multiple congenital defects. One hundred million viable organisms of *E. coli* were fed with the formula, after first demonstrating that this strain was not present in the infant's intestinal tract. Within 24 hours diarrhea and weight loss followed; the serotype D433 was found in small numbers in the throat and in large numbers in the feces and nasopharynx. When a different strain of *E. coli*, which was isolated from the infant prior to the experimental feeding, was similarly fed, no ill effects followed.

June, Ferguson, and Worfel (10) reviewed the literature concerning feeding of human volunteers. Ferguson and June (11) fed a mixture of three strains of *E. coli* 111B$_4$ in milk to adult volunteers. In these experiments with 114 volunteers, symptoms of acute bacterial food poisoning occurred when dosages of several million organisms were fed. An example of severe illness involved an adult volunteer fed 6,500,000,000 *E. coli* 111B$_4$ organisms at 3:00 P.M., who, by evening, complained of loss of appetite, unusual fulness, and gas. Sometime after midnight the patient passed 7 watery stools, 2 of which were cultured and found positive for *E. coli* 111B$_4$. The patient complained of urgency and tenesmus, and the following morning he vomited once. Nausea, stomach-ache, extreme fatigue, and occasional cramps were observed. There were 2 watery stools in the afternoon and 5 watery stools and cramps in the evening. However, by that time the appetite was slightly improved, although cramps were occasionally noted up to the sixth day, when the patient fully recovered. In one experiment where 9,000,000,000 *E. coli* 111B₄ were fed to each of 12 volunteers, 3 severe, 7 moderate, and 2 slight illnesses resulted.

A large percentage of the volunteers who ingested *E. coli* 111B₄ developed serum agglutinins, some without manifesting symptoms. Those volunteers who ingested a strain of *E. coli* isolated from a normal infant had no symptoms, nor did agglutinins develop in their sera to the strain fed.

June, Ferguson, and Worfel (10) fed adult human volunteers a mixture of three strains of *E. coli* 55B₅ in milk in an experiment involving 71 persons. The volunteers experienced symptoms ranging from a mild gastrointestinal upset to a severe gastroenteritis similar to acute food poisoning. The severity of the symptoms corresponded to the dosage fed, and no bacteremia was observed. The symptom complex was milder than that produced with *E. coli* 111B₄ organisms of comparable dosage. The symptoms and signs considered diagnostic were abnormal stools, emesis, abdominal cramps, nausea, flatulence, anorexia, headache, hyperpyrexia, insomnia, weakness, and lassitude. Below a level of 1,700,000,000 organisms the disease response was slight and the incubation period erratic. Again, volunteers ingesting *E. coli* from a normal infant neither developed symptoms nor showed significant rise in serum agglutinins. Volunteers who ingested killed *E. coli* 55B₅ organisms experienced no ill effects traceable to that organism and exhibited no rise in agglutinins.

The illnesses caused by feeding large doses of strains of *E. coli* 111B₄ and 55B₅ were, in general, mild. Fever in those made ill was commonly present from 18 to 20 hours after feeding. The organisms were not isolated from the blood or urine in any volunteers or in adults from throat specimens. Rubenstein and Britten (12) pointed out that epidemic diarrhea of infants is not limited to newly born infants but may affect older children and also occur among adults in the community.

It is interesting to note that the pathogenic strains of *E. coli* appear to be widespread in the United States and Europe. It is important in evaluating the significance of an agent in gastrointestinal illnesses to make certain that other agents which may cause diarrhea are excluded. Lindberg, Young, Belnap, and Warren (13) made careful tests for virus agents in the stool specimens submitted from infants with diarrhea from the Fort Belvoir outbreak. No viruses were found, and *E. coli* 0111 was isolated. No other enteric pathogenic bacteria were found by them.

The number of outbreaks of food poisoning which may be caused by specific strains of *E. coli* is unknown. Sera are not generally available for typing these strains, and they are often overlooked by diagnostic laboratories. The ease with which these organisms may be spread is pointed out by Rogers (14) in a study which he made in a cubicled ward, in which cases occurred. He states:

> The dust from the floor, the bath, the plug that went into the bath, the table used whilst the baby was being fed, the cot side, blankets and sheets, toys, the thermometer and the powder in the nursing chair of each child, the cracks where the window panes are sealed into the metal framework, the ledge on which notes were rested and the hand-towel used to wipe the hands of anybody handling a baby, were all heavily contaminated with the type strains of *Bact. coli.*

With such dissemination, it is not difficult to see how some of these coli types might find their way into food. Although data are available on the dosage of *E. coli* 0111B$_4$ and 055B$_5$ required to cause illness in adults, no information is available for infants and children. It is probable that smaller dosages are effective in causing illness for the younger age groups.

Escherichia coli has many times been associated with outbreaks of food poisoning, but there is no definite proof, except for the specific types indicated, that this organism is the responsible agent. Lodenkämper (15) has reviewed the literature and reported outbreaks of food poisoning which he believes are caused by *E. coli.* His evidence is based on the search for the causative organisms on Endo's medium and for toxins in broth. Tests for a toxin were made by oral and intraperitoneal injections into mice. This type of evidence is not conclusive, as was discussed previously under *Salmonella.* Plating on Endo's medium is unsatisfactory for detecting staphylococci and streptococci, which therefore may be missed.

Savage (16) makes the following statements in regard to the role which intestinal bacteria play in food-poisoning outbreaks:

> In the first place massive bacterial infection with intestinal bacteria is exceedingly common and foods such as milk, ice cream, brawn and sausages are habitually consumed containing thousands of bacteria per cubic centimeter or gramme, many of which are of direct intestinal origin. Food poisoning outbreaks should be of repeated and constant occurrence instead of being comparatively infrequent.

In another place he writes:

> We have finally the impressive fact that the more carefully and fully individual outbreaks are studied and bacteriologically investigated the greater the number found to be associated with infection with some definite bacillus, and it is a reasonable assumption that the residuum of outbreaks unassociated in this way would be comparatively small if all were fully investigated, bacteriologically and chemically, and especially if material was available for examination early in the course of the outbreak.

PARACOLON ORGANISMS

The paracolon organisms form a large group of heterogeneous coli-like organisms which have physiological characteristics unlike typical *Escherichia*. Taxonomically, some workers (17) have considered them intermediate between the typical coliforms and the *Salmonella*. In a small outbreak of gastroenteritis (18) a subgroup of these organisms was isolated from stool and rectal swab specimens from 17 of 52 patients. The implicated food—corn pudding—was not available for laboratory study. The incubation period averaged 12 hours, and the symptoms in the 52 cases were characterized by diarrhea (92.3 per cent), abdominal cramps (75 per cent), nausea (50 per cent), and vomiting (11.5 per cent). Recovery was complete in 12 hours. No tests were made for a-type streptococci, since none of the food in question was available.

One group of organisms in the paracolon group, designated the "Arizona group," is defined as follows:

> Motile rods which produce H_2S but fail to form indole; are methyl-red positive and Voges-Proskauer negative; produce acid and gas from glucose; do not utilize d-tartrate when tested by the method of Brown, Duncan and Henry or ferment sucrose, dulcitol or salicin; ferment lactose with varying avidity and slowly liquefy gelatin. Grow on Simmon's citrate agar [19].

These organisms produce fatal infections in reptiles, fowls, and lower mammals. In man they have been associated with cases of gastroenteritis and have been isolated from the blood and organs of fatal infections at necropsy.

Murphy and Morris (20) described two food-borne outbreaks caused by the "Arizona group" of enteric bacilli. The first outbreak involved 6 Negro children. The source of infection was apparently from a picnic lunch eaten at about 5:00 P.M. Nausea and vomiting developed, and in 2 cases chills and headache occurred. The children were admitted to the hospital with diarrhea, dehydration, and fever varying from 103° to 105° F., with one child reaching 107° F. shortly after admission. Temperature returned to normal in 2 or 3 days. Goose-liver sandwiches and ice cream were the foods common to all. Goose-liver sausage was excluded, since a specimen was examined and no pathogenic organisms were found. Furthermore, more people had eaten the sausage without becoming ill. The ice cream was home-made, but, since none was available for laboratory tests, no clues were found as to how it became contaminated.

The second outbreak occurred in a tuberculosis hospital involving 6 white male patients ranging from nineteen to forty-five years of age. Less than 24 hours preceding the onset of illness the patients had been served a special mixture consisting of milk, raw eggs, chocolate, and malt powder. The employee who had prepared the food was recovering from diarrhea of 3 days' duration. Positive stool specimens were obtained from him and from 3 of the 6 patients. Agglutinins were found in the sera from the patients with greater frequency and in higher titer than was observed among a control group which was not infected.

Attention has been given the "Arizona group" of paracolon bacteria as pathogens of animals and probably man by Edwards, West, and Bruner (21). This group was first studied by Caldwell and Ryerson (22) in strains isolated from horned lizards, Gila monsters, and chuckawalla. The strains were first classified as *Salmonella arizona* with the formula XXXIII:z_4, z_{23}, z_{26} . . . but are now considered paracolon bacteria. Seligmann, Saphra, and Wassermann (23) found an identical culture in the feces of a woman affected with fever, vomiting, and diarrhea. Edwards *et al.* (21) studied a culture from an infant affected with colitis.

The Bethesda-Ballerup group of paracolon bacteria has been associated with outbreaks of diarrhea. Edwards, West, and Bruner (21) studied 32 strains from 4 outbreaks of diarrhea. Subsequently, West and Edwards (24) combined the Bethesda and Ballerup groups of paracolon bacteria because of the similarity in biochemical properties and numerous serologic relationships between the two groups. They drew no conclusions concerning the role of the organisms in the production of enteric disease on account of their frequent occurrence in the intestinal tract of apparently normal persons and animals.

CLOACAE-AEROGENES GROUP

Early in 1930 an outbreak of gastroenteritis attributed to cream-filled pastry occurred in an area of 20 square miles in New York and New Jersey (25). In every case, the symptoms were said to have been manifested within a few hours after eating either cream puffs or chocolate éclairs made by a wholesale bakery. About 125 cases developed on 2 successive days. *Staphylococcus aureus,* found in large numbers in the cream filling, was excluded by the authors, because animal-inoculation tests were negative. Thus 5 ml. of a 48-hour culture grown in medium containing ingredients similar to those used in the pastry filling failed to cause symptoms when fed to a monkey. A guinea pig and a mouse were inoculated intraperitoneally with 2 and 1 ml., respectively, of a filtrate from the culture. Two rabbits were inoculated intravenously with 3 ml. of either this filtrate or one from a broth culture. None of the animals showed evidence of illness. An organism belonging to the cloacae-aerogenes group was thought to be responsible, since it was isolated from 5 fecal specimens and from the filling of 5 cream puffs or éclairs. The growth products of this organism proved toxic for certain animals. This outbreak, with its short incubation period, was, however, in all probability due to staphylococci, since it is obvious that the foregoing tests did not exclude staphylococcus food poisoning. As shown previously, the monkey is extremely resistant to the enterotoxin as compared to man. Mice, guinea pigs, and rabbits are unaffected by the parenteral injection of enterotoxin. Similarly, such animals are unaffected by the injection of boiled filtrates. When filtrates are boiled, the other toxins are greatly weakened or destroyed, but the staphylococcal enterotoxin is not appreciably affected. It cannot be emphasized too strongly that filtrates of cultures of the common Gram-negative intestinal bacteria may be toxic when injected into animals and yet be without effect when fed to man (26).

Proteus

Proteus vulgaris has frequently been associated with food poisoning. An outbreak was reported in Bristol, England (27), after brawn had been eaten which was thought to be contaminated with toxin produced by organisms of the *Proteus* group. The evidence was based on the intraperitoneal injection of kittens with filtrates prepared from cultures grown overnight on semisolid agar in 10 per cent carbon dioxide. Evidence of this type is valueless, since it has not been established that the intestinal tract is permeable to the toxic agent which is demonstrated by parenteral injection.

In this country an outbreak of food poisoning involving 34 people was traced to smoked fish (28). No specific food-poisoning organisms were isolated, but bacteriological examination of several samples of the fish revealed high bacterial counts, with *Proteus* predominating. No proof was brought forth, however, to show that *Proteus* was responsible for the food poisoning.

In an outbreak of food poisoning traced to sausage (29), about 2,000 soldiers were affected. Illness was characterized by vomiting, diarrhea, and exhaustion. In most cases symptoms appeared 2–3 hours after eating. A low-grade fever occurred in only the severe cases, which promptly subsided following treatment. Two hundred soldiers were hospitalized. Those who did not eat sausage were not ill, nor were those who had eaten from the same shipment of sausage 2 days earlier. A bacteriological examination of sausage revealed cocci and *P. vulgaris*. No *Salmonella* was found. The symptoms were those of staphylococcus food poisoning, although *Proteus* was listed as the causative agent, since it occurred before staphylococcus food poisoning was generally recognized.

Proteus mirabilis was thought to have a probable etiologic relationship in an outbreak of food poisoning in the navy traced to baked ham (30). In this instance 29 cases were reported; and 19 were hospitalized. Symptoms were severe and consisted of nausea, vomiting, and diarrhea, and their onset averaged 3 hours after eating. Of 19 hospitalized, 3 had passed blood, 16 had abdominal cramps, and 3 had fever with a maximum of 101° F. Sixteen had normal or subnormal temperatures. *Proteus mirabilis* was isolated from suspected ham and from 9 of 19 patients studied. A bacteriological examination of the ham revealed 62,000 organisms per gram, of which 12,000 per gram were staphylococci. Staphylococcus food poisoning was considered unlikely because of the low count of these organisms. No record was given as to whether the ham had been kept at a warm temperature for a number of hours before cooking. Under these conditions the heat-stable staphylococcus enterotoxin would still be present after cooking, although the organisms would be killed.

Proteus organisms are common inhabitants of the intestinal tract of man and animals. The numbers of these organisms may be, but usually are not, markedly increased when intestinal function is impaired. In a study of the isolated colon of a patient (31) with an end-ileostomy, *Proteus* organisms were frequently encountered at times when the colon was in a healing phase. In one period of 112 days, during which oxygen insufflation of the colon was carried out, 43 bacteriological examinations were made, and it was observed that *Proteus* colonies appeared in large numbers only during short periods of improvement of the colon. It has been the author's experience that, in patients with chronic ulcerative colitis, when the colon was acutely involved in exacerbations of the disease, *Proteus* was usually absent, whereas, during periods of remission, *Proteus* was often found in large numbers.

Proteus organisms are commonly found in large numbers in the feces of *Macaca mulatta*. Many appeared in the isolated colon of one of these animals (32). However, when 10 ml. of defibrinated sterile sheep blood was injected daily into the isolated colon, *Proteus* colonies were absent after 2 weeks and did not reappear until $4\frac{1}{2}$ weeks later, although daily blood injections were given over a period of 55 days.

An outbreak (33) of food poisoning involving 180 persons was traced to the meat from a hog which had showed evidence of septicemia at the time of slaughter. *Proteus* and colon bacilli were found in large numbers in the meat, but, by using selective media, *Salmonella* organisms were recovered. Since *Salmonella* organisms were found in the stools of patients and specific agglutinins were found in the serum, *Proteus* and colon bacilli were excluded as possible causative agents.

Savage (16) has reviewed the literature on 9 outbreaks of food poisoning attributed to *Proteus* and concluded: "From this summary of outbreaks it is evident that for none of them was it established that *B. proteus* was etiologically concerned."

Proteus is commonly encountered in the intestinal tract of man and animals who are not suffering from food poisoning. Its frequent occurrence when food poisoning is not concerned must, therefore, be explained if it is to be given etiological significance in food poisoning.

The Providence group appears in many ways to be intermediate between enteric bacteria resembling *P. morgani* and *P. rettgeri* but differs from these *Proteus* species in certain important aspects, such as failure to hydrolize urea. The Providence group has been associated with urinary-tract infections and has been commonly found in the stools in small outbreaks of diarrhea, as well as in the stools of healthy individuals. This group has been studied by Stuart and co-workers (34) and by Ewing, Tanner, and Dennard (35). Furthermore, the Providence group, made up of Gram-negative bacteria, is in the Enterobacteriaceae family. These bacteria produce acid in glucose within 24 hours, giving rise to a small amount of gas. Lactose is not fermented. Most cultures utilize sucrose after a long incubation, while mannitol is not fermented. Adonitol is used by most cultures. Indole is produced, growth occurs on Simmons' citrate agar, and the methyl red reaction is positive. Acetylmethylcarbinol is not formed, urea is not rapidly decomposed, and hydrogen sulphide is not formed in Kligler's agar or triple sugar iron agar. Most members of this group are motile.

Clostridium perfringens (*welchii*)

In England and Wales for the years 1941–48 (36) a total of 6 outbreaks was reported in which the presumed causal agent was *Clostridium perfringens*. In 1949 (37) it was reported that in a few outbreaks the causative organism appeared to be a heat-resistant strain of *Cl. perfringens*. In 1950 (38) 24 outbreaks were reported, and in 1951 and 1952 (39) 20 outbreaks, or 5 per cent of the total, were reported for each year. Of the incidents attributed to *Cl. perfringens*, 87 per cent were associated with processed, made-up or canned meats, or gravy stock.

Glynn (40) found no harmful results from ingesting cultures of *Cl. perfringens*. This bacillus was reported in the stools of patients in epidemics of diarrhea, but, since it is ubiquitous and commonly found in feces, its causative role was not definitely established. *Clostridium perfringens* is present in soil, water, milk, dust, sewage, and the intestinal canal of man and animals (41). It has been shown to be present in commercial "bread starters" for salt-rising bread (42).

In view of these circumstances the role of *Cl. perfringens* in outbreaks of gastrointestinal illness has been slow in being recognized. An outbreak of illness in children characterized by fluid stools with an offensive odor and by fever was outlined by Nelson (43). In these cases the abdomen was acutely distended by gas in the intestinal tract, and pus was present in the stools. The milk which these children received was found to be heavily contaminated with *Cl. perfringens*, and when a noncontaminated acid milk was fed, the diarrhea and abdominal distention promptly subsided, and the stools became normal. This rapid change to normal by merely changing the food suggests that the symptoms were due to an active fermentation process in the intestinal tract with mechanical distention of the bowel giving rise to nausea and hyperperistalsis.

Hobbs *et al.* (44) quoted Knox and MacDonald (1943) and Duncan (1944) as drawing attention to the possibility of an anaerobic spore-bearing bacterium causing outbreaks of food poisoning, Knox and MacDonald described illnesses in school children from meals prepared in a central kitchen. Gravy made on the previous day was found to be heavily contaminated with anaerobic spore-bearing bacilli. Duncan described outbreaks of diarrhea in residents of a wartime camp who had eaten meat and potato pie containing large numbers of *Cl. bifermentans*.

McClung (45) described 4 outbreaks in which chickens were cooked by steam under low pressure for a period of 3 hours, then removed from the broth and boned, the broth being saved for later use. The fowl was cooked on the day previous to serving. He suggested that the organism survived the heating temperature and grew in the broth during the storage period. The food item implicated was creamed chicken croquettes prepared from the cooked chicken and browned in deep fat. The symptoms were characterized by nausea, vomiting (rare), intestinal cramps, and pronounced diarrhea. In the majority of cases the symptoms began 8–12 hours after the meal, with the diarrhea continuing for about 12 hours. The following day most of those ill were able to continue normal activities. In McClung's studies *Cl. perfringens* was the only type of microorganism found in significant numbers. He suggested that a toxin might be responsible for the illness.

Zeissler and Rassfeld-Sternberg (46) studied strains of *Cl. per-*

fringens isolated from 1947 to 1949 from cases of hemorrhagic enteritis (enteritis necroticans, "Darmbrand") occurring in northern Germany. Several hours after eating tinned meat, rabbit, or fish paste, the patients developed low abdominal pain and diarrhea. In the severe cases the stools contained sloughed mucosa and blood, and deaths occurred from dehydration and circulatory failure. Where edema of the intestinal mucosa was severe, obstruction of the bowel developed. Large numbers of *Cl. perfringens* were present in the stools and in the lesions. Zeissler and Rassfeld-Sternberg differentiated the strains from *Cl. perfringens* type A on the basis of greater heat resistance. Spores of type A in nature are reported to survive 100° C. up to 90 minutes but, when grown in liver broth or brain pulp, they seldom resist boiling for more than 10 minutes. All strains of Zeissler and Rassfeld-Sternberg were found to resist boiling in the latter media for from 1 to 4 hours. On the basis of heat resistance these strains were designated type F.

Hormann and Schroeder (47) examined 52 soil and sewage samples taken from the areas of Hamburg, Lübeck, and Goslar and found *Cl. perfringens* type F in 26. Willich (48) examined 127 samples from stool specimens, duodenal secretion, intestinal loops, and 1 exudate of the abdominal cavity. Forty-one samples originated from 32 cases of illness. In almost all those in which the clinical and pathological anatomical diagnosis for enteritis necroticans was positive, *Cl. perfringens* type F was found. Hain (49) related finding *Cl. perfringens type* F in two cans of rabbit meat and one can of goose giblets. He reported that home canning of meat by cooking for 2 hours without pressure is insufficient to kill spores of *Cl. perfringens* type F. Hain searched for the organism in the intestines of persons not ill with jejunitis necroticans. Type F was estimated to be present in about one-sixth of the population of Hamburg during the winter of 1947 and 1948.

Cravitz and Gillmore (50) reported that nausea and cramps were evoked in 1 person and nausea and emesis in 4 from a group of 6 people fed 75–100 ml. of a heated (95° C. for 1 hour) filtrate of *Cl. perfringens*. The results were irregular in 9 others fed 50 ml. or less of the heated filtrate. The symptoms in these experiments appeared in 45–80 minutes after the filtrates were swallowed.

Hobbs *et al.* (44), whose studies began in 1946, described outbreaks of food poisoning suspected to be due to *Cl. perfringens*. From September, 1949, to February, 1952, 23 outbreaks were studied in which the supposed agent was heat-resistant *Cl. perfringens*. The food involved was usually meat, cooked and prepared the day before being eaten, and cooled slowly overnight. Ordinarily, no abnormal odor or flavor is observed. The symptoms follow an incubation period of 8–22 hours after mealtime and are characterized by acute abdominal pain and diarrhea; nausea and vomiting are rare. Chills, fever, headache, and other signs of infection are usually absent. The illness is short, lasting from a few hours to a day. In small family outbreaks the entire family may be affected, whereas in larger institutional outbreaks from 6 to 95 per cent of a group may become ill. In the experience of Hobbs and her co-workers the stools of patients or people involved are more likely to contain heat-resistant *Cl. perfringens* than the stools of those who are not.

In a study of the method of isolation of *Cl. perfringens*, Hobbs *et al.* (44) recommended the use of anaerobic blood agar plates incubated at 37° C. for 18 hours. Isolation is simplified when, after incubation, the anaerobic plate is left under atmospheric conditions at room temperature for 24 hours. This permits the aerobic organisms to develop, and the colonies of anaerobes can be more easily recognized. *Clostridium perfringens* is nonhemolytic. The implicated food specimen should not be heated prior to plating. On the other hand, where stools are examined, it is recommended that a pea-sized sample of stool be placed in broth and steamed for 1 hour, after which the suspension should be incubated anaerobically overnight and then plated on blood agar. The blood agar plates are incubated at 37° C. for 18 hours under anaerobic conditions.

Hobbs *et al.* (44) studied the toxins produced by these strains of *Cl. perfringens* and found them to be atypical from type A in producing only feeble alpha toxin, unable to produce theta toxin, variable in hyaluronidase production, and producing spores of greater heat resistance. These variations are not considered sufficient to separate them from type A strains. More work is needed to differentiate them from type F. In one outbreak the sera of 17 out of 32 patients possessed more than 0.005 unit of alpha antitoxin; in no case was beta or epsilon antitoxin found. The strains produce a Nagler reaction (lecithinase), which is inhibited by *Cl. perfringens* type A antitoxin. Eight serological types have been demonstrated by agglutination tests which cross-react serologically with some type A strains but have no relation to types B, C, D, E, and F.

Human volunteer experiments.—McClung (45) reported an illness in a volunteer who developed symptoms typical of those occurring in an outbreak after the volunteer had eaten a sample of chicken known to be contaminated with *Cl. perfringens*. Hobbs *et al.* (44) carried out several feeding experiments with human volunteers. One of these, fed 3 ml. of the supernatant fluid from a food-poisoning strain of *Cl. perfringens* grown in cooked-meat medium overnight, failed to develop symptoms. The culture was taken in milk. Another who swallowed 20 ml. of a 24-hour cooked-meat culture of strain 3702 developed abdominal pain and diarrhea 15 hours later, followed in $2\frac{1}{2}$ hours by further abdominal cramping. A man and a woman who were fed the same strain received a 10–15-ml. culture grown in Robertson's cooked-meat medium for 18–20 hours. Approximately 12 hours after taking the culture, one of the volunteers developed pain in the upper abdomen. Temperature was normal; abdominal pain increased intermittently and gradually diminished in intensity. Severe diarrhea occurred over the next 2 hours, also complaints of slight abdominal pain, headache, and nausea without vomiting. A second attack of diarrhea followed, with the volunteer unable to work for 1 day, after which recovery was rapid. The second volunteer had slight abdominal pain $14\frac{1}{2}$ hours after swallowing the culture but had no further symptoms. A volunteer fed a Seitz filtrate of a similar culture developed no illness; neither did volunteers fed a broth culture without meat or washed cells from a cooked-meat culture of the same strain.

Österling (51) fed human volunteers food from a hospital outbreak in which 583 of 1,034 people developed mild diarrhea 12 hours after eating. One individual who ate "pike perch" developed abdominal pain and diarrhea. No organoleptic changes were observed in the fish. Österling made a bacteriological examination of the fish and found no aerobes but observed *Cl. perfringens*. A fresh pike was dressed, cut up, and cooked, and 1 ml. of a 24-hour culture of the strain of *Cl. perfringens* isolated from the incriminated fish was injected deep into the muscle tissue. The fish was then held at

37° C. overnight, and pieces were fed the next day to 3 persons. Ten, 11, and 12 hours later, all three became ill with abdominal cramps and diarrhea, which lasted 10–12 hours. A volunteer who ate a portion from the same fish which was not inoculated with *Cl. perfringens* was not affected. Portions of the inoculated fish were macerated with a diluent and filtered. Three volunteers who received 10-, 25-, and 40-ml. amounts of the sterile filtrate did not become ill.

Feeding tests on monkeys, cats, dogs, pigs, guinea pigs, and mice with foods or broth inoculated with *Cl. perfringens* showed no clearcut reactions.

Österling (51) described another outbreak caused by *Cl. perfringens*. Over half of 60 people developed diarrhea, with an incubation onset of 12 hours after eating "veal head cheese" with an abnormal, sour smell. The head cheese contained a hemolytic bacillus and *Cl. perfringens*. Freshly prepared veal head cheese was inoculated with the hemolytic bacillus, incubated overnight at 37° C., and fed to a volunteer without causing illness. However, when the same freshly prepared veal head cheese was inoculated with *Cl. perfringens,* similarly incubated, and fed to a volunteer, 16 hours later illness with mild diarrhea that persisted for 8 hours resulted. In a later test a volunteer who ate veal head cheese inoculated with *Cl. perfringens* became ill in 13 hours. Volunteers fed steak sauce and boiled beef inoculated with *Cl. perfringens* and incubated overnight at 37° C. also became ill. In a 2-year period Österling (51), who studied 33 food-poisoning outbreaks, found *Cl. perfringens* to be the predominating organism in 15 outbreaks. In only 2 of these were the foods (meats) organoleptically abnormal.

Dack *et al.* (52) fed 21 volunteers, in amounts varying from 100 to 150 ml. each, filtrates prepared from four actively growing 24-hour veal-infusion broth cultures of *Cl. perfringens*. Each filtrate was mixed with 150–200 ml. of milk. No abdominal cramps or diarrhea developed. Where 200 ml. of the entire veal-infusion broth cultures in milk were fed to 20 volunteers, no illness resulted. Twelve volunteers fed 250 ml. each of autoclaved chicken broth inoculated with *Cl. perfringens* and incubated for 30 hours at 37° C. in anaerobic jars failed to develop symptoms. Hobbs (53) studied the 4 Mc-Clung strains which Dack *et al.* (52) fed. Serologically, 3 of them were not types 1–10, and 1 was a nonhemolytic type 7.

Information is needed to explain the role of *Cl. Perfringens* as a causative agent in outbreaks of food poisoning. Hobbs *et al.* (44), Österling (51), and Dack *et al.* (52) failed to cause symptoms in human volunteers fed filtrates of cultures of *Cl. perfringens*. Hobbs *et al.* (44) caused illness in volunteers fed whole-meat cultures of *Cl. perfringens*. Österling (51) caused illness in volunteers fed foods freshly prepared, inoculated with suitable strains of *Cl. perfringens*, and incubated overnight. Dack *et al.* (52) failed to cause illness in volunteers fed whole veal-infusion broth cultures in milk or whole chicken broth cultures of *Cl. perfringens*. Hobbs (53) suggested that these negative results may be due to the absence of whole meat in the cultures. Further work with human volunteers is necessary to elucidate the mechanism of the mode of action of *Cl. perfringens* in causing illness.

Bacillus cereus

Outbreaks of food poisoning have been attributed to spore-forming Gram-positive aerobic bacilli which were found in implicated food items. Hauge (54), a veterinarian in Oslo, Norway, carefully studied several outbreaks in which *Bacillus cereus* was the causative agent. These illnesses were characterized by an incubation period varying from 8 to 16 hours but more often from 12 to 13 hours. The symptoms were nausea, sometimes vomiting, and severe cramplike abdominal pains in the lower part of the abdomen and around the umbilicus. Tenesmus and cramplike contractions of the rectum occurred without defecation. However, watery diarrhea was common in many cases, with the passage of 4–6 stools. Usually the illness was over in 6–12 hours and was not accompanied by fever or weakness.

Hauge studied four large outbreaks involving 600 persons. Three of these outbreaks occurred in hospitals, and 1 in a home for aged people. In one instance, vanilla sauce prepared from a commercial powder was involved. A sauce was made from some of the stock powder to simulate the outbreak. The sauce was stored for 1 day at room temperature under conditions identical with those preceding the outbreak. A plate count after 24 hours revealed 36,000,000 *B. cereus* per milliliter. By direct microscopic examination, 100,000,-000–110,000,000 *B. cereus* per milliliter were found. Hauge ate 200 ml. of the sauce and 13 hours later developed severe abdominal pain, tenesmus, and frequent watery stools. There was no fever or generalized weakness, and he recovered in 8 hours.

Potato and corn starch are considered to be naturally contaminated with *B. cereus*. Hauge warns against keeping foods prepared with these starches at favorable incubation temperatures for a time before they are served. Six human volunteers were fed from 155 to 270 ml. of vanilla sauce containing from 30,000,000 to 60,000,000 *B. cereus* per milliliter. Two of the subjects were unaffected, 2 became slightly ill, and 2 developed pronounced symptoms. Stool examinations revealed either an absence of *B. cereus* or only a few organisms.

Christiansen, Koch, and Madelung (55) described an outbreak in a summer camp in Marseliborg, where 15 out of 18 adults and 106 out of 130 children (between eight and sixteen years of age) became ill after eating a meal containing yellow pudding. The pudding had been stored in cups for 24 hours at a temperature favorable for bacterial growth. Cultures revealed 13,000,000 *B. cereus* per gram; no other bacterium appeared on the plates. The symptoms were similar to those described by Hauge, and other causative agents were excluded.

Dack, Sugiyama, Owens, and Kirsner (52) fed washed cells of either whole milk cultures or whole vanilla sauce cultures of *B. cereus* to 47 human volunteers. Of 5 volunteers fed 8,400,000,000 washed cells of *B. cereus*, 1 had a loose stool 12 hours after feeding and no other complaints. None of 5 fed 10,400,000,000 viable *B. cereus* in milk was ill; nor were 6 volunteers fed whole vanilla sauce cultures containing 5,150,000,000 viable *B. cereus* ill. Laboratory strains of *B. cereus* which were fed gave the same biochemical reactions that Hauge described for his strains. It is regrettable that the *B. cereus* strains isolated by him were not available for this study. More work is needed to explain the failure to duplicate Hauge's work with *B. cereus*.

UNIDENTIFIED AGENTS

A vigilant search for new causative agents of food poisoning should be maintained, but caution should be exercised in multiplying the number of microbial agents on the basis of presumptive, inconclusive evidence (56). Year after year some of the same agents are reported in the literature without additional proof as to their etiological significance.

REFERENCES

1. JORDAN, EDWIN O., and IRONS, ERNEST E. J. Infect. Dis., 11:21–43, 1912.
2. ———. *Ibid.*, 13:16–29, 1913.
3. BRAY, J. J. Path. & Bact., 57:239–47, 1945.
4. GILES, C., and SANGSTER, G. J. Hyg., 46:1–9, 1948.
5. GILES, C., SANGSTER, G., and SMITH, J. Arch. Dis. Childhood, 24:45–53, 1949.
6. TAYLOR, J., POWELL, B. W., and WRIGHT, J. Brit. M. J., 2:117–25, 1949.
7. KAUFFMANN, F. J. Immunol., 57:71, 1947.
8. SMITH, J., GALLOWAY, W. H., and SPEIRS, A. L. J. Hyg., 48:472–83, 1950.
9. NETER, ERWIN, WEBB, CHARLES R., SHUMWAY, CLARE N., and MURDOCK, MIRIAM R. Am. J. Pub. Health, 41:1490–96, 1951.
10. JUNE, R. C., FERGUSON, W. W., and WORFEL, M. T. Am. J. Hyg., 57:222–36, 1953.
11. FERGUSON, W. W., and JUNE, R. C. Am. J. Hyg., 55:155–69, 1952.
12. RUBENSTEIN, A. DANIEL, and BRITTEN, SIDNEY A. J. Pediat., 38:457–62, 1951.
13. LINDBERG, R. B., YOUNG, V. M., BELNAP, W. D., and WARREN, J. Paper presented at annual meeting of A.P.H.A. in Buffalo, 1954.
14. ROGERS, K. B. J. Hyg., 49:140–51, 1951.
15. LODENKÄMPER, H. Centralbl. f. Bakt., Abt. 1, 145:306–14, 1940.
16. SAVAGE, W. G. Food poisoning and food infections. Cambridge: At the University Press, 1920.
17. STUART, C. A., and RUSTIGIAN, ROBERT. Am. J. Pub. Health, 33:1323–25, 1943.
18. BARNES, L. A., and CHERRY, W. B. Am. J. Pub. Health, 36:481–83, 1946.
19. KAUFFMANN, F. Enterobacteriaceae. Copenhagen: Ejnar Munksgaard, 1951.
20. MURPHY, W. J., and MORRIS, JANIE F. J. Infect. Dis., 86:255–59, 1950.
21. EDWARDS, P. R., WEST, MARY G., and BRUNER, D. W. Kentucky Agr. Exper. Stat. Bull. 499, April, 1947.
22. CALDWELL, MARY E., and RYERSON, DWIGHT L. J. Infect. Dis., 65:242–45, 1939.
23. SELIGMANN, E., SAPHRA, I., and WASSERMANN, M. Am. J. Hyg., 40:227–31, 1944.
24. WEST, MARY G., and EDWARDS, PHILIP R. Public Health Monogr. No. 22. Washington: U.S. Dept. Health, Education and Welfare, 1954.
25. GILBERT, RUTH, COLEMAN, MARION B., and LAVIANO, ALICE B. Am. J. Pub. Health, 22:721–26, 1932.
26. DACK, GAIL M., CARY, WILLIAM E., and HARMON, PAUL H. J. Prevent. Med., 2:479–83, 1928.

27. COOPER, K. E., DAVIES, JOAN, and WISEMAN, JEAN. J. Path. & Bact., **52**:91–98, 1941.
28. KLEEMAN, IRVING, FRANT, SAMUEL, and ABRAHAMSON, ABRAHAM E. Am. J. Pub. Health, **32**:151–58, 1942.
29. BAERTHLEIN, K. München. med. Wchnschr., **69**:155–56, 1922.
30. CHERRY, W. B., LENTZ, P. L., and BARNES, L. A. Am. J. Pub. Health, **36**:484–88, 1946.
31. DACK, G. M., and DRAGSTEDT, LESTER R. Am. J. Digest. Dis., **5**:84–86, 1938.
32. DACK, G. M., DRAGSTEDT, LESTER R., and HEINZ, THEODORE E. J. Infect. Dis., **60**:335–55, 1937.
33. SCHÖNBERG, F. Ztschr. Fleisch- u. Milchhyg., **54**:82, 1943.
34. STUART, C. A., WHEELER, K. M., and McGANN, V. J. Bact., **52**:431–38, 1946.
35. EWING, W. H., TANNER, K. E., and DENNARD, D. A. J. Infect. Dis., **94**:134–40, 1954.
36. Month. Bull. Min. Health, **9**:148, 1950.
37. *Ibid.*, p. 254.
38. *Ibid.*, **10**:228, 1951.
39. *Ibid.*, **13**:12, 1954.
40. GLYNN, E. E. 1915. Cited by SIMONDS, J. P. Monogr. Rockefeller Inst. M. Res. No. 5, September 27, 1915.
41. WILSON, G. S., and MILES, A. A. Topley and Wilson's The principles of bacteriology and immunity, **1**:886. 3d ed. Baltimore: Williams & Wilkins Co. 1946.
42. KOSER, STEWART A. J. Infect. Dis., **32**:208–19, 1923.
43. NELSON, C. I. J. Infect. Dis., **52**:89–93, 1933.
44. HOBBS, BETTY C., SMITH, MURIEL E., OAKLEY, C. L., WARRACK, G. HARRIET, and CRUICKSHANK, J. C. J. Hyg., **51**:75–101, 1953.
45. McCLUNG, L. S. J. Bact., **50**:229–31, 1945.
46. ZEISSLER, J., and RASSFELD-STERNBERG, L. Brit. M. J., **1**:267–69, 1949.
47. HORMANN, HARWIG, and SCHROEDER, WALTER. Deutsche med. Wchnschr., **74**:749, 1949.
48. WILLICH, GERT. Deutsche med. Wchnschr., **74**:1339–40, 1949.
49. HAIN, ERNST. Zentralbl. Bakt., Abt. I Orig., **153**:315–22, 1949.
50. CRAVITZ, LEO, and GILLMORE, JAMES. *Clostridium perfringens* in human food poisoning. Unpublished report presented at 78th annual meeting of A.P.H.A., October 31, 1950.
51. ÖSTERLING, SVEN. Nord. hyg. tidskr., **33**:173–80, 1952.
52. DACK, G. M., SUGIYAMA, H., OWENS, FRANCIS J., and KIRSNER, JOSEPH B. J. Infect. Dis., **94**:34–38, 1954.
53. HOBBS, BETTY. Personal communication.
54. HAUGE, STEINAR. Nord. hyg. tidskr., **31**:189, 1950.
55. CHRISTIANSEN, O., KOCH, SVEND O., and MADELUNG, P. Nord. med., **3**:194–202, 1951.
56. DACK, G. M. Am. J. Pub. Health, **37**:360–64, 1947.

IX *Infections To Be Differentiated from Food Poisoning*

There are many infections which may simulate food poisoning and give rise to diarrhea, abdominal cramping, nausea (with or without vomiting), and pyrexia. These infections must be ruled out, however, in dealing with food poisoning, and no detailed explanation will be given about them. Yet, as previously discussed, there is one outstanding difference. Food poisoning, in its inception, is generally of an explosive nature, whereas epidemics of infectious disease may break out over a period of several days.

BACILLARY DYSENTERY

Upon several occasions the author has been called upon to investigate apparent outbreaks of food poisoning which were later found to be bacillary dysentery. Although much has been written about this disease and many infectious agents have been described, little is known of the natural habitat of the organism. Man is a natural host for bacillary dysentery, while *Shigella*, which is pathogenic for man, has never been reported in domestic animals which furnish meat for food. In areas in which typhoid fever and cholera are controlled, bacillary dysentery remains endemic. It is common where groups of people are housed together, as, for example, in prisons, asylums, armies, and among populations in summer-resort areas. Selective media have been devised for the isolation of dysentery bacilli from feces, but it is well known that during convalescence the organisms often disappear rapidly from the stools and are undetectable even with the most selective laboratory methods. The fact that bacillary dysentery is universal indicates that there are many undetected carriers. This contention is justified in experiments with the monkey (*Macaca mulatta*), which is a natural host for Flexner dysentery bacilli. Although these microörganisms may not be recovered through the best technical procedures from the stools of these monkeys, the animals spontaneously develop the disease (1, 2, 3) when placed on vitamin-deficient diets.

Shaughnessy and his co-workers (4), in testing the effectiveness of vaccines for bacillary dysentery, challenged human volunteers with freshly isolated strains of *Shigella paradysenteriae* (Flexner W).[1] They fed 100,000,000 living organisms in milk to 4 unvaccinated persons without producing diarrhea or fever. In a second group of 4 volunteers who received 1,000,000,000 living organisms of the same strain fed in milk, none developed temperature. One patient passed four watery stools on the second day after he had drunk the culture. In both groups positive stool cultures occurred within 48 hours. In a third group none of 4 subjects showed elevated temperatures when fed 10,000,000,000 living organisms of the same strain in milk. A fourth group of 4 volunteers received 10,000,000,-000 living organisms of the same strain in water. Three of this group of 4 were ill, and the fourth experienced slight cramps. The 3 made ill experienced cramps within a few hours after the dysentery bacilli were swallowed. Two had frequent watery stools. The third patient vomited and had severe cramps up until the tenth day after inoculation. In a fifth group 15,000,000,000 organisms of the same strain were fed in water to 4 subjects, and none showed any signs or symptoms during the next 24 hours. They were then given an additional 15,000,000,000 on each of the following 2 days without effect. On the fourth day, 50,000,000,000 more organisms were given, and only mild headache, anorexia, slight abdominal cramps, and an occasional soft stool resulted.

In addition to these tests, some volunteers were fed human feces infected with the same strain of *S. paradysenteriae,* and others were fed more recently isolated strains. Of 30 volunteers who received no vaccine and who were fed living *Shigella* cultures, only 19 developed dysentery. The incubation period in the experimental disease, with few exceptions, was no longer than 24 hours. A strain of *Shigella* virulent for Swiss mice when injected intraperitoneally failed to produce clinical infection in man, while other strains of much lower

1. Each volunteer received 1 drachm (4 ml.) of paregoric 3½ hours after a meal, followed ½ hour later by 2 gm. of powdered sodium bicarbonate in 1 ounce of water. After 5 minutes the dysentery bacilli, suspended in ½ pint of milk or, in later experiments, in a glass of water were given.

virulence for mice produced severe dysentery. These experiments illustrate the variability of the susceptibility of man to infection and the importance of the virulence of the organism in producing infection. Furthermore, the fallacy of attempting to evaluate the pathogenicity of these organisms for man on the basis of parenteral injections into other animal species is well shown. This experimental study with *Shigella* parallels closely some of the results obtained in similar studies with *Salmonella*.

Bacillary dysentery may be spread by food contaminated with feces from carriers or from sufferers from the disease. In any outbreak, however, the cases appear over a period of days rather than within a short space of time. This difference, together with the recovery of the bacilli from stools by culture, is sufficient to differentiate the disease from food poisoning. It is recommended that cultures of stools be made in all cases in which bacillary dysentery is suspected.

INFECTIOUS HEPATITIS

One form of infectious hepatitis may be food-borne. This type, caused by a virus, has an incubation period of from 10 to 40 days, or an average of 25 days. The disease is characterized by the following symptoms: anorexia, general malaise, fatigability, headache, nausea, chills and fever, vomiting, and upper-right abdominal tenderness. Jaundice may or may not be present.

Capps and Stokes (5) pointed out that experimental transmission of the disease has been accomplished by both the parenteral and the fecal oral routes. Through the use of adult volunteers it was shown that a fecal carrier state of from 5 to 15 months may occur. More information is needed concerning the duration of the carrier state.

Read *et al.* (6) described a food-borne outbreak of infectious hepatitis in a fraternity house. In most cases the onset of the disease was insidious. Malaise, general myalgia, chills, fever, and, in addition, anorexia appeared early and became severe after 4–7 days. In many cases almost intractable vomiting occurred. Dark urine was noticed soon after the onset of the illness. By the fourth or fifth day, fever began to subside, and jaundice followed. In this outbreak between May 26 and June 5, 1944, 24 cases occurred. Of 101 fraternity members, 14 lived and ate their meals in the house. Four cases developed in this group, constituting an attack rate of 28.5 per cent. Of 60 men eating all or part of their meals at the house, 20 were affected, an attack rate of 33.3 per cent. Of the remaining 27 members who ate only an occasional meal at the house, none became ill. No cases occurred in students outside the fraternity, even though the members had contact with other students. Spirochetal jaundice was excluded.

Kaufmann *et al.* (7) reported an outbreak of viral hepatitis in which 14 cases appeared within from 23 to 36 days after a cook in a battery mess contracted the disease. The role of personal contact could not be disproved in this outbreak, yet contaminated food was strongly suspected as the vehicle of infection.

AMEBIC DYSENTERY

Amebic dysentery may occur in epidemics, as demonstrated at the Century of Progress Fair in Chicago in 1933 (8). Amebic dysentery generally occurs sporadically and may continue to arise over a long period of time. The water-borne Chicago epidemic was shown to occur in individuals staying at certain hotels in which the plumbing was faulty and a back siphonage of sewage occurred in the water lines. The disease may also be food-borne. Usually, amebic dysentery is endemic and spreads by intimate personal contact. It is differentiated from food poisoning by being of an insidious and chronic nature. The incubation period from the time of ingestion of the amebae to the onset of symptoms may vary from less than 1 week to 4 months in a few cases. The attacks range from mild intermittent diarrhea to an acute fulminating type of bloody flux. Many of the people apparently acquiring the infection during the Chicago epidemic did not develop symptoms until some time after they had returned to their homes in other parts of the country. *Endamoeba histolytica*, the causative agent of amebic dysentery, should always be excluded before making a diagnosis of food poisoning, especially if only a few cases are involved. Detailed methods have been devised for the laboratory diagnosis of this protozoan (9, 10). Its presence in stools should be interpreted with caution, however, as approximately 10 per cent of the population are infected, and the majority of these suffer no noticeable symptoms.

TRICHINOSIS

The early stages of trichinosis have been confused with food poisoning. Some years ago the author was consulted about some cases in which, since several people died, physicians were considering the diagnosis of botulism. Each member of an Italian family concerned in the outbreak developed acute diarrhea. At necropsy of two of the children who died, larvae of *Trichinella spiralis* were seen in abundance in the muscle. An inquiry into this outbreak revealed the source of the infection. The father had brought home a dead hog found on a dump, from which sausage was made without cooking. The meat was found to contain numerous encysted larvae.

Trichinosis is caused by a nematode, *T. spiralis,* which man usually acquires from insufficiently cooked, infected hog meat. A description of this infection may be found in textbooks on parasitology. When encysted larvae are eaten, the cysts are digested in the patient's stomach, whereupon the larvae excyst in the duodenum. They invade the duodenal and jejunal mucosa and give rise to symptoms such as nausea, vomiting, diarrhea, dysentery, colic, and profuse sweating. It is in this stage of the infection, about 48 hours after ingestion of the larvae, that the disease must be differentiated from food poisoning. If a history of the eating of uncooked or improperly cooked pork is known, encysted nematodes may be sought in the food, if available. There is no practical method for excluding trichina from pork at the time of slaughter, but thorough cooking removes the danger of infection. As the disease progresses, the diagnosis becomes more evident. When the larvae migrate into the tissues, patients may develop a severe myositis, spastic paralysis of the muscles, and edema of the face and hands.

Diagnosis depends upon the stage of the disease. A marked eosinophilia is suggestive of trichinosis. During the intestinal phases, adult worms are sometimes recovered from the feces. During and after larval migration, the larvae are often found in muscle strips removed at biopsy. Various modifications of Bachman's (11) intradermal and precipitin tests with worm extracts are valuable, especially in the later stages of trichinosis.

EPIDEMICS OF ACUTE DIGESTIVE UPSETS OF VIRAL OR OF
UNKNOWN ETIOLOGY

Dingle and his associates (12), in studying common illnesses occurring over a period of 3 years in 292 individuals in 61 families in the Cleveland, Ohio, area, found that gastrointestinal illnesses were second in frequency after respiratory infections. In their work they reported that gastrointestinal illnesses were comprised chiefly of acute nonbacterial gastroenteritis.

Epidemics of acute digestive upsets which cannot be associated with food or water have been reported in widely scattered localities (13). In an outbreak of 41 cases (13), the onset was mostly gradual, beginning with nausea, vomiting, and diarrhea. The patients became ill over a period of hours. In some individuals it was associated with colds, but in many there was no history of any upper respiratory infection. In 29 cases where symptoms were tabulated, diarrhea, the most common, occurred in 25, nausea in 20, vomiting in 23 (the second 2 most common), and fever in 13. Some of the ambulatory patients were ill for only a few hours, whereas others were ill from 2 to 3 days. There was some evidence that illness was spread by contact or possibly by droplet infection, since it was limited to certain floors in one dormitory and to 2 individuals, who had contact with those ill, who were afflicted 4 days later. No intestinal pathogenic organisms were detected in fecal cultures. Furthermore, attempts to find a virus by inoculating monkeys (*M. mulatta*) intranasally with nasopharyngeal washings failed. Two monkeys injected intraperitoneally with citrated blood from 2 patients did not develop a nasal discharge or diarrhea. Inasmuch as this outbreak occurred over a period of several days and was not associated with food or water, it could readily be differentiated from food poisoning.

Goodall (15) reported an epidemic, around the end of January, 1953, in England, of "winter vomiting disease" which was characterized by a patient awakening in the early hours to throw up copiously. The vomiting was preceded by nausea, epigastric pain, and some collapse, followed by loose, pale stools. Nausea lasted for a day or two, after which recovery was complete. Dr. Goodall was not impressed with the infectivity of the disease, since, out of his 46 patients, there were 35 cases where only 1 individual in a household was affected. Of the group, 5 patients had an upper respiratory infection at the time of attack. Two of the 46 patients attributed their illness to food.

Reimann, Hodges, and Price (16) reported 2 epidemics of widespread mild disease, characterized by anorexia, malaise, diarrhea, nausea, and vomiting. These outbreaks, in October and November, 1943 and 1944, occurred in Philadelphia, its environs, and in other widely scattered places. Bacteriological study of the stools and pharyngeal secretions of 10 patients revealed no unusual bacteria or parasites to account for the disease. About 100 mice were injected intranasally, rectally, or orally with the supernatant fluid from centrifugation of diarrheal stool samples mixed with saline from 5 patients. Pharyngeal washings in bouillon were inoculated intranasally into mice and, after filtration, intracerebrally. Some mice developed a pneumonitis, and further lung passages were carried out in some to the fourth serial passage. From these studies no virus was isolated. Intranasal inoculations of stool filtrates into 8 four-week-old calves were also negative.

Reimann and his associates (17) then resorted to experimentation on student volunteers. Suspensions of diarrheal stools and broth garglings were passed through a Mandler filter. The resulting filtrates were nebulized and passed into a large box into which the volunteer placed his head for 5 minutes. Of 21 students inhaling nebulized stool filtrates, 11 developed typical diarrheal symptoms after an incubation period of less than 4 days. In 3 cases the diarrhea was accompanied by a mild nasopharyngitis. Of 32 students who inhaled nebulized filtered garglings, 17 developed diarrhea without nasopharyngitis. No symptoms developed in 6 who inhaled nebulized patient's serum. A group of 15 students swallowed 3 ml. of filtered garglings in double gelatin capsules. Five swallowed stool filtrates and 4 patients' sera similarly encapsuled. No symptoms followed this oral administration. Since these investigations were carried out during the course of a natural epidemic without precautions for isolation, further work is necessary to evaluate the results properly.

In contrast to the work of Reimann and his associates is that of Gordon *et al.* (18), who studied an epidemic disease in several New York State institutions. The illness was characterized clinically by sudden onset, profuse diarrhea, usually vomiting, and often cramps, headache, and dizziness. Fever was slight or absent, and no characteristic bacterial agents could be demonstrated. Recovery followed within 48–72 hours, although in some cases 1 week was required. Respiratory symptoms were not evident. Experiments were reported with 28 human volunteers. All subjects were kept under hospital isolation in isolation cubicles. Human volunteers fed fecal filtrates in capsules from cases of epidemic gastroenteritis developed gastroenteritis. The incubation period ranged from 1 to 5 days, or a mean of 3 days. The disease was carried through three generations, in the last two by means of fecal filtrates. Oral administration of unfiltered throat washings from experimental cases of the disease induced gastroenteritis, although subjects inhaling a portion of the same throat washings remained asymptomatic. Embryonated hens' eggs were inoculated with one unfiltered stool suspension that had been used in a pool with another stool suspension which had induced gastroenteritis when fed to each of 3 volunteers. Three sets of eggs were inoculated; one on the chorio-allantoic membrane, another into the yolk sac, and a third into the amniotic sac. Streptomycin and penicillin were used as antibacterial agents. After three serial passages by each method, tissue and extra-embryonic fluids were noninfective for volunteers.

Subsequently, Gordon and his associates extended their work. One outbreak was studied in Rockland State Hospital, New York (19), where 913 cases occurred in 9 weeks, with an attack rate of 15 per cent of the population. In this outbreak the patients were housed in different buildings, and the peak of the epidemic varied for the separate structures. In each housing unit illness occurred over a period of several days, and the cases were not correlated with an age or sex difference. No evidence was found to incriminate the water or milk supply.

Gordon *et al.* (20) studied the blood, urine, and spinal fluid in volunteers made ill after being fed the infectious agent causing the nonfebrile disease. No abnormalities were found.

Jordan, Gordon, and Dorrance (21) compared the reactions in human volunteers of an infectious agent, F.S., from the stools of a patient in the Family Study in Cleveland (12), with the Marcy strain originally isolated from an institutional outbreak in New

York. The Marcy strain, which usually produces an afebrile illness, with an average incubation period of 60 hours, is characterized by watery diarrhea. The F.S. strain, with an average incubation period of 27 hours, produces a febrile illness and is characterized by constitutional symptoms, with usually normal or loose stools. Jordan *et al.* believed that the two agents were different, since, in addition to clinical variations, there is no cross-immunity. Intranasal instillation of throat washings obtained from two cases of gastroenteritis failed to produce illness in two volunteer groups.

Kojima *et al.* (22) and Yamamoto *et al.* (23) transmitted afebrile gastroenteritis occurring in Japan to human volunteers by fecal specimens from cases of nonbacterial gastroenteritis. These investigators confirmed Gordon's work with the Marcy strain but did not study the cross-immunity of the strains.

The prodigious amount of excellent work by Dr. Irving Gordon and his associates has demonstrated beyond a doubt that infectious agents are in stools during the acute stage of gastrointestinal illnesses where no pathogenic bacterial agents have occurred. Resistance to the infectious agents follows recovery, and it remains for future studies to determine how long immunity lasts. At least two agents have been recognized, and perhaps more may be subsequently discovered. As Dr. Gordon has frequently pointed out, a simple laboratory test is needed for the recognition of these agents. Although naturally occurring outbreaks of nonamebic, nonbacterial enteritis do not appear to be food-borne, food cannot be excluded as a vehicle of infection until more is known of the causative agents and their ability to survive in nature outside the host.

Smillie, Howitt, and Denison (24) studied an epidemic of acute watery diarrhea occurring in Jefferson County, Alabama. The incubation period for 40 cases based on known contact ranged from 1 to 12 days, with a median of 3 days. Environmental sanitation was good; water, food, and milk did not appear to be sources of infection. The length of illness ranged from 1 to 14 days, with 5.1 days the mean. There was no age group exempt, and both men and women were attacked equally. Numerous attempts were made to isolate a virus by various methods in both embryonated eggs and small animals, but no virus was found from either fecal specimens or nasal washings.

Although many outbreaks of epidemic diarrhea and vomiting are reported (25, 26, 27), there is reason to believe that the vast majority are unrecognized. Since this type of infection simulates the symptoms of food poisoning, it is important that the two be differentiated. A striking difference is that epidemic diarrhea has not been related to food or water and that an epidemic in a community may cover a period of many weeks. Certainly, it is of the utmost importance to exclude these illnesses from the category of food-poisoning outbreaks.

CONCLUDING REMARKS

Symptomatology, epidemiology, and pathology are all essential and must be included in establishing a correct diagnosis and intelligent analysis of any outbreak of food poisoning. Where these data are not considered and evaluated, specific agents may be falsely incriminated. In this book a critical discussion is given of the various agents which may cause food poisoning, and it is hoped that the similarities and distinctions which have been drawn will prove helpful to individuals engaged in studying the numerous gastrointestinal upsets which may be due to food poisoning.

REFERENCES

1. VERDER, A. E., and PETRAN, E. J. Infect. Dis., **60**:193, 1937.
2. TOPPING, N. H., and FRASER, H. F. Pub. Health Rep., **54**:11, 416, 1939.
3. JANOTA, MARTHA, and DACK, G. M. J. Infect. Dis., **65**:219–24, 1939.
4. SHAUGHNESSY, HOWARD J., OLSSON, ROLAND C., BASS, KENNETH, FRIEWER, FRANCES, and LEVINSON, SIDNEY O. J.A.M.A., **132**:362–68, 1946.
5. CAPPS, RICHARD B., and STOKES, JOSEPH, JR. J.A.M.A., **149**:557–61, 1952.
6. READ, MARGARET R., BANCROFT, HULDAH, DOULL, JAMES A., and PARKER, ROBERT F. Am. J. Pub. Health, **36**:367–70, 1946.
7. KAUFMANN, GUSTAV G., SBOROV, VICTOR M., and HAVENS, W. PAUL. J.A.M.A., **149**:993–95, 1952.
8. Nat. Inst. Health Bull. 166, March, 1936.
9. TONNEY, FRED O., McILHENNY, MARIAN, HOEFT, GERALD L., and KOONG, C. H. Canad. Pub. Health J., **26**:335–48, 1935.
10. Am. Pub. Health A. Year Book, pp. 130–43, 1935–36.
11. BACHMAN, GEORGE W. J. Prevent. Med., **2**:35, 513–23, 1928.
12. DINGLE, J. H., BADGER, G. F., FELLER, A. E., HODGES, R. G., JORDAN, W. S., JR., and RAMMELKAMP, C. H., JR. Am. J. Hyg., **58**:16–30, 1953.
13. GRAY, J. D. Brit. M. J., **1**:209–11, 1939.
14. DACK, G. M. Am. J. Digest. Dis., **8**:210–11, 1941.

234 *Food Poisoning*

15. GOODALL, JOHN F. Brit. M. J., **1**:197–98, 1954.
16. REIMANN, HOBART A., HODGES, JOHN H., and PRICE, ALISON H. J.A.M.A., **127**:1–6, 1945.
17. REIMANN, H. A., PRICE, A. H., and HODGES, J. H. Proc. Soc. Exper. Biol. & Med., **59**:8–9, 1945.
18. GORDON, I., INGRAHAM, H. S., and KORNS, R. F. J. Exper. Med., **86**: 409–22, 1947.
19. GORDON, IRVING, INGRAHAM, HOLLIS S., KORNS, ROBERT F., and TRUSSEL, RAY E. New York State J. Med., **49**:1918–20, 1949.
20. GORDON, IRVING, MENEELY, J. K., JR., CURRIE, GORDON D., and CHICOINE, ALICE. J. Lab. & Clin. Med., **41**:133–41, 1953.
21. JORDAN, WILLIAM S., JR., GORDON, IRVING, and DORRANCE, WILLIAM R. J. Exper. Med., **98**:461–75, 1953.
22. KOJIMA, S., FUKUMI, H., KUSAMA, H., YAMAMOTO, S., SUZUKI, S., UCHIDA, T., ISHIMARU, T., OKA, T., KURETANI, K., OHMURA, K., NISHIKAWA, F., FUJIMOTO, S., FUJITA, K., NAKANO, A., and SUNAKAWA, S. Jap. M. J., **1**:467, 1948.
23. YAMAMOTO, A., ZENNYOJI, H., YANAGITA, K., and KATO, S. Jap. M. J., **1**:379, 1948.
24. SMILLIE, JOHN W., HOWITT, BEATRICE F., and DENISON, G. A. Pub. Health Rep., **63**:233–43, 1948.
25. BROWN, G., CRAWFORD, G. J., and STENT, LOIS. Brit. M. J., **1**:524–26, 1945.
26. HARGREAVES, E. R. Brit. M. J., **1**:720–22, 1947.
27. POND, M. ALLEN, and HATHAWAY, JOHN S. Am. J. Pub. Health, **37**: 1402–6, 1947.

Index

235

PRINTED IN U.S.A.